Traditional Chinese Qigong for Health

Traditional Chinese Qigong for Health

Chan Siok Fong

authorHOUSE®

AuthorHouse™ UK Ltd.
1663 Liberty Drive
Bloomington, IN 47403 USA
www.authorhouse.co.uk
Phone: 0800.197.4150

Published by AuthorHouse 06/14/2013

ISBN: 978-1-4817-8758-1 (sc)
ISBN: 978-1-4817-8759-8 (hc)
ISBN: 978-1-4817-8760-4 (e)

For my daughter, Jeng.

To my niece, Quan, my sister, Sook,
my brother, Hoe, and all my relatives
and friends.

In memory of my deceased brother, Loon,
who, during his lifetime, patiently accompanied
me to the gardens.

An Important Note to All Readers

Today's world is busy and tense. People tend to take the easy way to try out different ways and means to self-heal. Though this book is predominantly a work on "self-aid to self-cure", it is not intended as a substitute for professional medical advice for any of your ailments, be they chronic or acute. Do not let this book prompt you into using it first for self-healing, ignoring the real need for medical diagnosis of your illnesses. Use the ideas given in the book to complement professional medical guidance in a common quest for better health.

The author accepts no responsibility for the results of your efforts and will not be liable for any loss or damage that arises from information, ideas, and experiences provided in this book.

Contents

About the Author

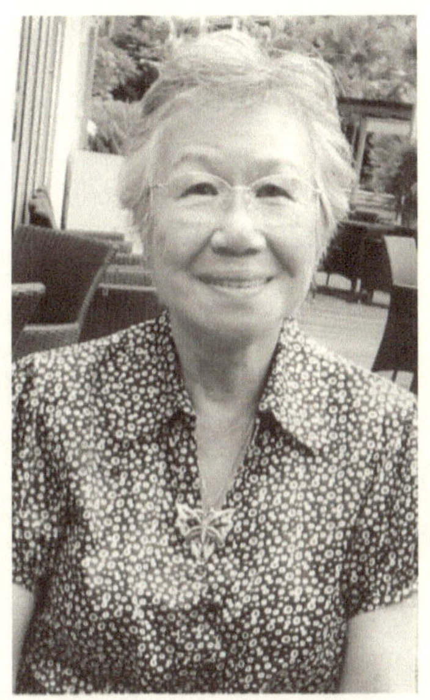

Chan Siok Fong
M.Ed. in Educational Studies (Sheffield)

By profession, Chan Siok Fong is a retired school teacher from Singapore. Due to the poor health she suffered from childhood through adulthood, she reached the point in 1986 where she decided to seek healing from Traditional Chinese Qigong (TCQ). After two years, people who had known her previously and were aware of her general weakness were amazed by the change in her general well-being and her increased energy levels. After twenty-six years of constant Qigong practice, the benefits she gained in her health cannot be questioned, and now at the age of seventy-nine she has decided to share her knowledge and experience with others by writing this book.

Author's Health and Her Association with Traditional Chinese Qigong

My Health

I was never healthy through the years from childhood to adulthood. Now that I am seventy-nine going on to eighty, I still carry with me the living memory of the years of inner despair at not being able to receive appropriate treatment for my chronic ailments, pains, and aches. However, the twenty-six years during which I have put into use the Traditional Chinese Qigong practice has been the unforgettable happiest episode of my life.

Since having a bout of measles at the age of three in 1936—I was told I nearly died of it—I was never in good health. As far as I can remember, from 1942 all the way into the 1950s, my vulnerability to respiratory infection, constant fever, pain and swelling of the joints, muscle spasms, and the deformity of my left knee were of no serious concern to the adults. The family's western-trained doctor did not think I was suffering from rheumatoid arthritis. She fed me with antibiotics whenever respiratory infections set in, but she ignored my joint pain and constant muscle cramps.

In school I played several types of games and took on numerous activities to keep myself busy enough to forget the depressing aches and pains.

During adulthood, from the 1950s through the 1980s, when I was working long hours and living a stressful lifestyle, my pains worsened. I consulted several western-trained medical doctors about my cervical spondylosis, endometritis, chronic gastric problem with hyperacidity, and stomach ulcer. All the doctors recommended surgery. I declined surgery and resorted to taking the drugs the doctors prescribed. As years went by, my ulcer was healed, but the tightness in my chest and at times palpitations and shortness of breath developed. Headache was a daily occurrence. From time to time my heart beat turned irregular. My blood pressure was low; the systolic pressure was seventy-five and the diastolic pressure was sixty. I consulted a heart specialist, and he recommended a pacemaker for the heart. I shuddered at the thought of electrical currents racing across my heart, and therefore I decided to live on with the ailments. A few years later, another heart specialist told me I had a rheumatic heart and nothing could be done. As for other ailments, each time I went to the doctor, I was given antibiotics, tranquillizers, and analgesics. My illness was taken for granted as just "semi-sick" discomforts.

As age advanced, more ailments set in—frozen shoulders, pain down the spine, swollen knees, and pain in the jaw joint. These pains were wearing me down. There were times when I used only an arm and a leg and my body would falter. At other times my knees would buckle, and I would find myself sliding down the stairs or falling flat on my face. Doctors diagnosed this as signs of an accelerated aging process. I was given pills, and then they changed the pills . . . added more . . . then scanning . . . testing . . . physiotherapy . . . traction . . . heat treatment . . . and finally they suggested the possibility of an operation. I asked myself what the consequences would be if I took the operation. What could be accomplished? Would continuation of modern medical treatments minimise the gravity of the degenerative conditions of the heart and stomach, would they cure the shortening of muscle fibres, the tremors, and the pains?

My Association with Traditional Chinese Qigong (TCQ) Practice

In 1986 at the age of fifty-three, on the recommendation of the Chinese physician Mr Dai, whom I frequently consulted for herbal treatment, I left for China to take up Qigong lessons at the Shanghai Qigong Research Institute. I was assigned two eminent Qigong masters. Old Master Ma Ji Ren concentrated on teaching meditation. He lectured on history and basic concepts in relationship to Qigong practice. He also taught the initial method of "healthcare meditation"—how to sit correctly for a relaxed posture, how to exhale and inhale gently to achieve a slow, smooth, long, and deep breath, and how to calm the mind to cause the brain to be free of disturbing thoughts. Master Ma also taught a breathing exercise to resolve any shortness of breath encountered during meditation.

My second master was Shen He Nian who had spent years of research on "Cultivation of the Internal Qi" 《内气练养功》. He identified a form of mobile Qigong named "*Da Yan Liu Zi Gong* (大雁六字功)" for my chronic ailments. It consists of seven exercise regimens. Master Shen's laboratory investigations and clinical experiments had proved the effectiveness of this exercise for the proper functioning of the liver, heart, spleen, lungs and kidneys, and the lymphatic and endocrine systems.

My Diligent Practice

On returning home, I diligently gave myself a little practice each day, and each day I gained something new. The smooth flow of the *qi* and blood was manifested on my face. The pallid look vanished. I felt physically and mentally relaxed and emotionally stabilised. Pains and aches were reduced and I was not so vulnerable to infections. The tightness in my chest and rib cage, the pain, and the heart palpitations petered out. My blood pressure and cholesterol levels were regulated. I lost some weight, but the great change was in my general well-being and my balanced levels of energy, which gave me greater vitality and mental clarity. Friends who were aware of my previous health conditions were amazed at my improvement. I knew then that the danger level of my health had passed.

Years later in 2001, I returned to Master Shen He Nian in Shanghai for revision and sharing of the therapeutic effects of Qigong. Master Shen also shared the latest updates and upgrades and gave further lessons on how to regulate the breathing and calm the mind. The exercises provided special focus on relaxation. I also received lessons on how to self-massage with acupressure. At this final session, Master Shen gave helpful hints on how to use massage and acupressure on commonly used energy points as "self-aid" to treat the sudden occurrence of chronic pains and discomforts.

With this last session, my quest for a broad-based Traditional Chinese Qigong practice to resolve my chronic ailments ended. This course had given me adequate therapeutic support. Taking a step further, I immersed myself in books, reading everything I could about Traditional Chinese Qigong practice, and I picked up variables that could be adopted to maximize benefits for my health. Between the years 2001-2007, I also attended three international symposiums on Qigong science organised by the Shanghai Qigong Institute in Shanghai, China. My purpose in attending was to follow closely the latest developments in scientific research on Qigong cultivation. Theory and practice had enabled me to capture the basic concept of Qigong and its special characteristics and its visible effects on health.

In the years that followed, the evidence of Qigong's therapeutic effects was unquestionable. How Qigong resulted in helping me to resolve my ailments is difficult to explain; but it is something I felt inside me. The vital force of the healing energy *zhen qi* (真气) is ethereal. I just feel "right". Qigong certainly has therapeutic efficacy in strengthening my muscles, nerves, and bones, and it enables the visceral organs, the lymphatic and endocrine systems—in short, the whole body—to function normally.

With the feeling of wellness I derived from "healthcare meditation" I progressed into "oneness meditation". This systematic progression promotes further relaxation of the body, during which the mind becomes perfectly still, silent, and empty of emotions, egoistic thoughts, and prejudices. The breathing becomes naturally effortless. The balanced *yin-yang* (阴阳) force of the life-energy *qi* attained from the first thirty minutes of healthcare meditation continues to move forcefully, blending the body's "essence fluid 精", "energy force 气", and "spiritual consciousness 神" into a spiritual strength. The goal of oneness meditation is to conserve this spiritual strength and further develop it into achieving "oneness" of "body-mind-spirit" with nature's law. At this stage, the full potential of healthiness, a good-natured disposition, and a creative intelligence were unfolded, endowing upon me an all-in-one spiritual wisdom. This spiritual wisdom uncovers an awareness of a Higher Self in accord with a sense of seeing (having an insight into) the true nature of things. This insight has given me that extra sensitivity to spot signs of problems and deftness in listening to the body to detect which part of the body is in trouble and then adopt the right approach to cope with the malady. A step further is the ability to accept death as a natural phase in life—a *blissful way* to rest a cleansed soul.

Acknowledgements

First I wish to thank the 1986 Shanghai Qigong Research Institute of the University of Traditional Chinese Medicine in China for assigning two veteran Qigong masters as my tutors. Without my masters' generous sharing of skills and knowledge gained from their years of research and advancement with Traditional Chinese Qigong practice, I would not be around today to share my ideas and experiences with everyone. Herein my grateful thanks.

- Master Ma Ji Ren for his lectures on the historical and cultural impacts on the development of Qigong through the years; for his emphasis on the importance of knowing and understanding basic concepts in Qigong practice; and for lessons on "healthcare meditation".

- Master Shen He Nian for his untiring efforts in imparting his well-developed skills and knowledge of "*Da Yan Liu Zi Gong* (大雁六字功)" and massage with acupressure; for sharing his research knowledge on the effects of *qi* on health.

- I also wish to record here special thanks to my uncle, Chan Lai Kee of Malaysia, for sharing with me his skill in traditional massage and for introducing me to his collection of precious out-of-print books on massage and Traditional Chinese Qigong practice.

- The Art Sauce Studio of Singapore for the illustrations.

Introduction

This book describes how I recovered my health from a series of chronic ailments by means of Traditional Chinese Qigong practice. My friends have often asked me, "What is the meaning of the word Qigong?" and "What is Traditional Chinese Qigong?" Herein is the explanation.

Meaning of the Word "Qigong"

The word "Qigong" in Chinese is written in two ideograms as *qi-gong* (气 功). The first ideogram *qi* (气) refers to the energy *yuan qi* (元气), that is stored in the *dantian (丹田) elixir field* in the lower abdomen of our body, one and a half inches inward from the navel. *Yuan qi* (元气) is the inherent *qi* built from:

1. The oxygen and charged ions from the air we breathe in through natural exhalation and inhalation

2. The energy from the food we eat

3. The primordial energy

The second ideogram *gong* (功) means the art, skill, or technique applied to the practice of Qigong.

Traditional Chinese Qigong (TCQ)

Traditional Chinese Qigong has a history of about 2,500 years. It was started as a keep-fit activity. First it was realized that dancing could strengthen muscles, joints, and bones. Later on, some of the dances were developed into physical therapies for the treatment of heavy and sluggish limbs. As years went by, renowned Qigong masters decided to use the three basic theories founded in traditional Chinese medicine to guide their practices. They are the *yin-yang* (阴阳) theory, the energy *qi* channels经络 theory and the viscera脏腑 (internal organs) theory.

Qigong and the *Yin-Yang* (阴阳) Theory

The *yin-yang* (阴阳) theory is an ancient philosophical theory in traditional Chinese medicine healing that was adopted into Qigong practice by Qigong masters as a therapy for healthcare. It has been theorised that the inherent *yuan qi* (元气) in our body has two energy phases, the "*yin*" (阴) *phase* and the "*yang*" (阳) *phase*. Excess or deficiency of either phase in our body can affect our health. Too much *yin* (阴) energy will produce a cold (cooling) feeling, while too much *yang* (阳) energy generates a hot (heating) sensation. Energy we receive from the universe is *yang (阳)*, and energy from the earth is *yin (阴)*. The foods we eat also contain *yin (阴) and yang (阳)* energy. For example, bitter gourd has *yin (阴)*, and beef has *yang (阳)*. Eating too much of either food can upset our constitution; but if we eat the two together—for example, frying beef with bitter gourd—the actions of the food will balance the energy. Based on time-honoured records by renowned Chinese physicians, it is said that an unbalanced *yin-yang (阴 阳) qi* puts our body at risk of diseases if serious or of chronic discomforts if mild. This unbalanced condition has to be regulated in time; otherwise our health will suffer. Physicians used herbal medicine to correct the imbalance, and Qigong masters take into account a breathing technique. Thus, we see in Qigong practice, a long exhalation gets rid of excessive *yang (阳)* energy, while a long inhalation draws in more energy to tone up a *yin (阴)* constitution.

With additional studies on the *yin-yang (阳)* theory, modern scientific researchers on Qigong found that the inherent *yuan qi* (元气) has in it the *yin* and *yang* energy, containing positive and negative charges of electric current. They also confirmed *yin* (阴) (negative) and *yang* (阳) (positive) energy could become an electromagnetic force to transmute the inherent energy *yuan qi* (元气) into a vital life energy force *zhen qi* (真气) (subsequently written as *qi*) for healing. This *qi* can be activated to flow into the energy qi channels. Qigong practice in the form of meditation, mobile Qigong, or massage with acupressure has in it distinctive techniques to activate the *qi* to flow.

Qigong and the Energy *Qi* Channels Theory

Based on the theory of energy *qi* channels (经络) found in traditional Chinese medicine, Qigong research masters provided evidence of the existence of energy channels linking all parts of the body, with two main channels running down the midline—the front and back of the body trunk. Building on these facts, they developed techniques to regulate the body, the breath, and the mind to enable the *qi* to flow into the channels. Meditation is the main form used in Qigong practice to activate the *qi* to circulate. As the *qi* circulates, two functions are at work. The first is clearing the knots of energy clotted in the energy channels, giving rise to a smoother flow. With no blockages in its way, the *qi* becomes a force to pull along the nutrient-carrying blood cells to flow without difficulty into the blood vessels.

A common saying among traditional Chinese physicians and veteran Qigong masters is, "When *qi* flows, blood flows along." As blood carries nutrients to different parts of the body for nourishing and healing, the viscera theory of traditional Chinese medicine becomes another study by Qigong masters. They developed in Qigong practice a technique in directing the *qi* into the visceral organs, making it a safe therapy for health.

Qigong and the Viscera (脏腑) (Internal Organs) Theory

In traditional Chinese medicine, it is theorised that health depends on the strength and weakness of the *qi* that flow into the visceral organs—the liver, heart, spleen, lungs, and kidneys. When *qi* is depleted, diseases set in. When *qi* finishes, the functions of these organs cease. When *qi* circulates smoothly in a balanced manner, these organs are strengthened to function normally. Based on this theory, veteran Qigong masters designed sets of mobile exercises with fluid movements, "mind-will (意念)", and breathing disciplines to direct the *qi* to move into the visceral organs. The aim is to realize optimum benefits in procuring healthiness for the body.

The Seven Principles Governing Quality Qigong Practice

Based on the above three theories, veteran Qigong masters made further studies that resulted in the development of "seven principles" governing Qigong practice. Their goal is to bring about high-quality Qigong for all to abide by.

1. **Achieve relaxation and tranquillity naturally. (松静自然)**

   During Qigong practice *relaxation* means maintaining a good posture to relieve tension of muscles and nerves, and concentrating the mind to train the brain to be calm and restful, free of disturbing thoughts, and to allow breathing to become naturally slow and gentle. *Tranquillity* means the mind is in a perfect state of stillness, able to withstand internal emotional disturbances and external environmental irritations. In our Qigong practice, we move naturally from relaxation into tranquillity without any mental exertion or physical force. In this way we release ourselves from physical tension and mental stress. Body and mind will then be fully relaxed to allow a smooth flow of the *qi*.

2. **Include stillness and movement in a single practice. (静动相兼)**

   For Traditional Chinese Qigong to provide optimum conditions for health, every Qigong practice should combine stillness and movement. This means that in our daily practice, meditation (stillness) and mobile Qigong (movement) are best practiced together one after the other. In meditation, we maintain outward stillness to achieve inward restfulness to cause the internal *qi* to move out of the lower *dantian (丹田)* elixir field to circulate through the channels. We say there is internal activity when *qi* moves. In mobile Qigong, we adopt fluid movements of the limbs and body, mind-will (意念) and a breathing discipline to conduct the internal *qi* to circulate into the visceral organs. There is internal restful movement of the *qi* while our body is being externally active. Qigong masters maintain that this form of practice is a holistic approach to healthcare. Hence, we should involve both tranquil Qigong and mobile Qigong in any single practice session.

3. **Keep the upper part of the body void and maintain fullness at the lower part of the body** (上虛下实).

   Void at the upper part of the body means the head and chest should be relaxed so that the flow of *qi* is smooth. In Qigong practice, we breathe from the nose and allow the mind to direct the breathing down to the lower abdomen—sinking into the *dantian (丹田) elixir field*. We do not allow *qi* to amass at the head.

   Fullness at the lower part of the body means substantial *qi* is being stored at the lower abdomen dantian. To ensure the upper part of the body is void, we must never rest with *qi* stagnant at the head or chest. We must always remember to send the *qi* down to the lower abdomen before closing the exercise.

4. **Let '*mind-will* (意念) ' flow along with the breath (意气相随).**

At the start, mind-will (意念) is a mental activity concentrating with one thought to influence breathing in the movement of the *qi*. In Qigong practice, we use mind-will to train our breathing to be slow, smooth, long, and deep so as to move the *qi* out of the lower abdomen *dantian (丹田) elixir* field to circulate the *qi* channels. On reaching the highest degree of mind tranquillity, our *qi* will circulate on its own. By this time mind-will no longer exerts force on the breath to move the *qi*. It naturally follows the internal circulation of the *qi* without imposing any thoughts on the breath.

5. **Complement training with nurturing (练养相兼).**

Training means consciously regulating our breathing by mind-will at the lower abdomen to let it become slow, smooth, long, and deep. By concentrating at a specific location, stray thoughts are kept from disturbing the mind. *Nurturing* is to let go of all conscious regulation of breathing by mind-will. This means that during the nurturing stage, mind-will is no longer exerted on the breath. It interflows with the breath to allow it to strengthen the *qi* at the *dantian (丹田)* elixir field and to let it naturally move out of the *dantian (丹田)* into the *qi* channels. Practising training along with nurturing and vice versa is a form of practice that replenishes energy that may be lost during the exercise.

6. **Progress is made in stages (循序渐进).**

   Qigong exercises are not instant noodles. Each form of exercise has its own methodical techniques that require time to learn and to make progress step by step. Undue haste will unbalance the *yin-yang (阴阳)* energy in the *qi* and upset the *qi* flow. A disturbed flow is the origin of diseases. The essential step to good health is to maintain the equilibrium of the energy *qi* flow round our body visceral organs and systems. Only with regular and patient practice can we see good results.

7. **Return all *qi* to its root (引气归元).**

   The root is at *dantian (丹田)* elixir field in the lower abdomen where *qi* is stored. To obtain positive effects on health, after completing each phase of meditation, we ought to return the *qi* to its root by doing a "winding up" exercise. Refer to Section One (page 20-22)

   The above seven principles govern all forms of Qigong exercises. Practise well; the *qi* will strengthen the functions of our nervous system, respiratory system, digestive system, circulatory system, and internal secretion system to overcome chronic health conditions and recover our youthful vigour.

About This Book

My purpose in writing this book is to share with everybody, young and old, sick and well, the different forms of Qigong exercises that I have learnt and practiced for twenty-six years to regain my health. It contains useful information that provides knowledge and facts about the uniqueness of each Qigong practice. Each section has its own distinct areas, including proven and practical methods on how to prevent inaccurate practices. Hence, the purpose of this book is to bring readers to the point of knowing and understanding how to go about maintaining good health.

Section One highlights the practice of meditation to train and nurture the internal *qi* to provide healthcare and transcendental bliss with spiritual awakening. Section Two focuses on mobile Qigong, with a set of seven exercise regimens named *Da Yan Liu Zi Gong* (大雁六字功). In mobile Qigong, the mobility is capable of building and regulating the *qi* to pull the blood into the visceral organs, the lymphatic and endocrine systems, to improve their functions for healthy growth. Section Three provides a set of easy-to-manage massage with acupressure exercises. This has in it *qi* regulation functions that can give initial care for the sudden occurrence of pains and discomforts that result chiefly from work stress and an unhealthy lifestyle.

All the exercises have no religious or philosophical background. In order to appreciate Qigong practice, you should initially view it as a physical exercise to keep fit. As we go along, we will be interested in studying its effects in this regard and pursuing the exercises as a way of health for life. Sooner or later we will become conscious that with regular and constant practices, we are able to maintain our health at an acceptable level to overcome disease and premature aging.

It is my hope that this book and the essential TCQ exercises it describes will be like the key that opens the door for us to enter into living a healthier and longer life. It is also my wish to see everyone, irrespective of age, sex, culture, and physical condition, be inspired by the therapeutic potency of Qigong practice and not miss the chance to learn.

Section One

Meditation—A Tranquil Qigong
(静坐内养功)

An Exercise to Nurture the Internal *Qi*

Understanding Meditation

Brief History

More than 2,000 years ago, China's earliest medical collections, "*The Yellow Emperor's Canon of Internal Medicine* (黄帝内经), expounded upon a theory of Qigong methods and practices, including:

- "A mind that is calm and void (of thinking activities) enables '*zhen qi* (真气)' (vital life energy) to be realised." (恬惔虚无, 真气从之.)

- "Hold on to the inner strength of mind to keep sickness in check. (精神内守, 病安从来.)

- "The breath, the essence fluid, the energy force, and the preservation of spiritual consciousness single-mindedly keep muscles well coordinated." (呼吸精气, 独立守神, 肌肉若一).

After the Chinese Revolution of 1911, intellectuals advocated "meditative exercises" as a method to maintain good health. Representative works of that time were *Yin Shi Zi Meditation Methods* (因是子静坐法) by *Jiang Wei Qiao (蒋维乔), Essence in Meditation Exercises* (静坐法精义) by Ding Fu Bao (丁福保) , and *Methods for the Cultivation of Tranquility* (静的修养法) by Chen Qian Ming (陈乾明。) .

Since the founding of the People's Republic of China, Chinese medical physicians with Qigong knowledge, from 1978 onwards, have conducted extensive scientific research studies and clinical experiments to establish the effects of *qi* flow on health. They confirmed that during meditation, as *qi* flows and circulates the *qi* channels, the *qi* becomes a vital life force. This life force pulls the blood so that it flows and circulates smoothly in the blood vessels. Blood supplies the necessary nutrition, and *qi* the life-nourishing energy. Together they repair and heal damaged cells and tissues to prevent diseases and improve the immune system and brain function to cope with ailments and restore us to good health.

To this day, traditional Chinese medical physicians and Qigong masters have considered *qi* to be the source of life. Our health depends on the strength and weakness of the *qi*. When *qi* is depleted, diseases set in. When *qi* is exhausted, life ends. When *qi* flows and circulates smoothly in a balanced manner around the body, we feel well.

My Form of Meditation

From Healthcare to Oneness

Around us, we see meditation being practised by people in many forms for many different reasons. In my approach, based on the theoretical and practical lessons I received from Master Ma Ji Ren, and built on my twenty-six years of practical experiences, I settled for a three-phase approach from *healthcare* meditation into *oneness* meditation.

Healthcare meditation concentrates on nurturing the inherent *yuan qi* (元 气) to become a vital life energy *zhen qi* (真气) (subsequently referred as *qi*) that governs growth and health.

In oneness meditation, we progress from the healthcare state of quiescence into tranquillity to achieve "stillness" of the mind—"quieting the restlessness of the mind" (*Lao Zi's Dao-De-Jing* (道德经ca. 500BC). This stillness empties the mind of all distracting thoughts, ending all thoughts to move into a different dimension of the ultimate reality that is beyond time and space. In this state, the mind drifts into a deep level of "nothingness" to repose in a mystical union, a harmonious "oneness" with nature's law.

Over the years, this moment of "inner renewal" has given a second dimension to my life. There is this conscious self-awakening that leads to the unfolding of the latent creative intelligence. This creative energy is the energy of creativity and intelligence that surges to the brain (mind), enabling all mental confusion to be removed and allowing wisdom to surface instead. Most interestingly, there is this sixth-sense feeling that gives rise to the finest aspect of clear thinking, clear perception, and insight into every thought and action, enabling intuitive solutions to problems. This brings about significant improvements in performance without appearing busy. As mentioned in *LaoZi's Dao-De-Jing* (道德经), "Does nothing, yet there is nothing left undone (无为而无不为)." In today's society, it could be translated to mean "Minimum effort reaps maximum results."

ESSENTIAL ELEMENTS IN MEDITATION

The correct method of meditation involves knowing three essential elements that are prerequisites to all forms of meditation. These entail regulating the body for a relaxed posture; regulating the breath from natural and gentle to being slow, smooth, long, and deep; and regulating a disturbed mind to being calm and restful, eventually attaining quiescence and tranquillity.

For learners who are beginners, it is important to learn these essential elements correctly from the start, as they open up a significant prelude to subsequent practices on healthcare and oneness meditation.

Step I: Regulate the Body

In all forms of meditation, to regulate the body means to adopt a relaxed posture. This is important because mental and muscle relaxation reduce tension to give a soothing effect to the brain and the nerves. This soothing effect will eventually lead our mind into a state of calm and restfulness and cause our breathing to become natural and gentle.

There are different postures that we can adopt in my form of meditation. They include lying flat-back, standing straight, or sitting on a chair or stool. The choice should fit the individual's needs. Some people choose the standing posture, but in general the sitting posture is widely preferred. It is suitable for people of all ages. In all my practices, I adopt the sitting posture.

Different Postures

Figure 1: Lying Flat-Back

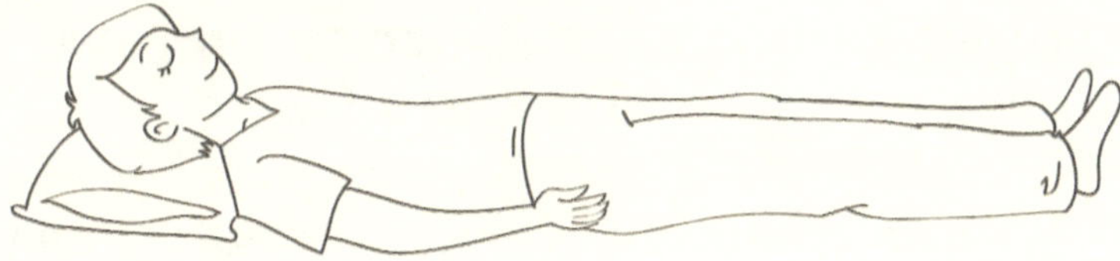

This lying down position is suitable for the elderly, the weak and the sick.

- Lie flat-back on a pillow of moderate height. Lightly close the eyes and mouth.

- Naturally stretch both arms with the elbows flexed and the hands by the sides of the body. Naturally stretch both legs with the feet apart to shoulder width or feet together with heels touching.

Figure 2: Natural Standing Posture

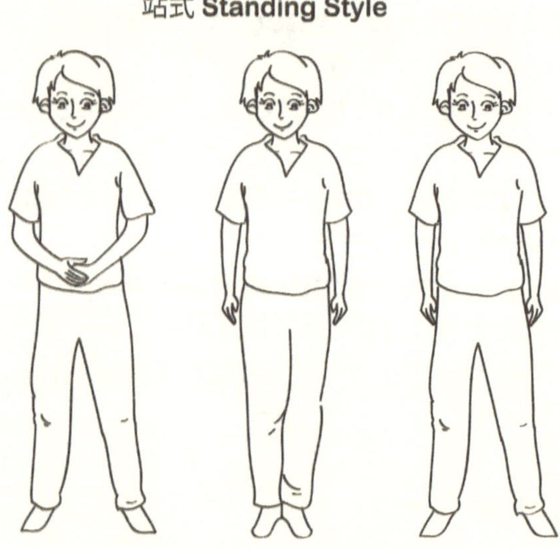

- Stand with feet together or feet apart to shoulder width with knees flexed.

- Hold your head comfortably erect. Keep your chin in by allowing your head to drop a little so that it is in a straight line with the neck. (Feel relaxed, not tight.)

- Relax the shoulders but do not hunch.

- Cup your palms one over the other (either left or right) on the navel in the lower abdomen.

- Lower your eyes to the ground or look horizontally at something pleasing to the eyes.

(Note: When lowering the eyes to the ground, drop the eyelids to the point of closing, but still remain able to see a thin stream of light.)

Figure 3: Sitting Posture

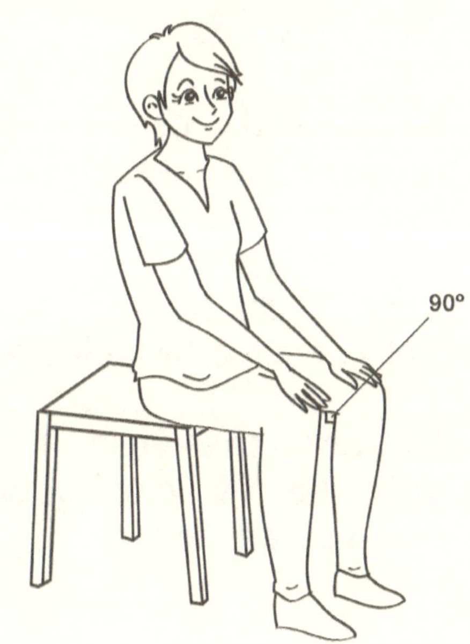

- Sit upright on a chair or stool. It should be high enough for you to put your feet firmly apart on the ground. Place your feet horizontally to the width of the shoulders.

The back of leg to the thigh should be at an angle of 90°.

- Having found your balance, hold yourself comfortably erect with your head and neck straight. Keep your chin in by allowing your head to drop a little to be in a straight line with the neck. (Feel relaxed, not tight.) Keep the tip of nose in a straight line with the navel.

- Relax your shoulders but do not hunch. The minor forward curve of the shoulders relaxes the chest and allows the energy to flow and circulate downwards.

- Rest the palms at a comfortable position on the lap or over the knees. Flex the elbows to avoid tensing up the arm muscles.

- Lower the eyes to the ground or look horizontally at something pleasing to the eyes.

(Note: When lowering the eyes to the ground, drop the eyelids to the point of closing, but still remain able to see a thin stream of light.)

Step II: Regulate the Breath

The breathing exercise is of the utmost importance in meditation. Our body needs the oxygen and charged ions from the air to bring about transformation of the inherent *yuan qi* (元气) into a vital life energy—the *zhen qi* (真气) for healing or the prevention of diseases. The smooth circulation of this vital life energy *qi* in the *qi* channels depends on the way we exhale (breathe out) and inhale (breathe in). In meditation, we generally exhale and inhale through the nose, unless specified otherwise. At the beginning, we aim for natural, gentle breathing. No force is used. Do not inhale fully; about ninety per cent should be enough. Do not exhale too quickly and violently. The final aim is to achieve a slow, smooth, long, and deep subtle breathing.

Method 1: Training for Natural and Gentle Breathing

With slightly opened lips, slowly and gently exhale through the mouth saying the word *soong (松)* meaning "relax". Then inhale lightly through the nose with the mouth closed, thinking of the word *jing* (静) meaning "quiet". Repeat this exercise nine times. Gradually drop the words and continue exhaling and inhaling naturally and gently through the nose for ten to fifteen minutes without exertion. Do this exercise every day until you feel comfortable and at ease. Then proceed to Method 2 on abdominal breathing.

(Note: If at the moment of practice our physical condition happens to be *yang* (阳) (feeling hot, discharging reddish yellow urine or hard stools), we do not hold the breath during the inhalation stage but give a long exhalation. If our physical condition is *yin* (阴) (feeling cold, having a pale complexion, discharging white urine or soft stools), we hold the breath longer and give a shorter exhalation. If our health is normal, we give equal time for exhalation and inhalation.)

Method 2: Training and Nurturing Abdominal Breathing

This training helps to strengthen the internal *qi* in the lower abdomen.

Concentrate on breathing slowly and gently at the navel in the lower abdomen. The concentration should be faint and the abdomen free from tension. This conscious resting of our thoughts and the slow and gentle breathing enable us to sense gradual movement in the abdomen. This is an indication that our breathing is deep. Some of us may sense the abdomen bulging out during inhalation and being drawn in during exhalation or vice versa, drawing in the abdomen upon inhaling and relaxing the abdomen (blowing it up slightly) upon exhaling. I leave it to my body to react. I do not pursue. As long as I feel comfortable and relaxed in my habitual way and the movement of the abdomen is comfortable, I carry on in that manner. Pay attention to the rise and fall movement of the abdomen for a minute or so. Then let go to move into the nurturing stage. Draw the thought away from the abdomen to just breathe naturally and quietly for as long as you wish. At any moment if the mind is filled with distracting thoughts, return to concentrating at the abdomen, and then let go again. Repeat these exchanges several times until you feel calm and restful.

(Note: Do this exercise every day for twenty minutes or more. After the exercise, stand up slowly. Take a slow walk for ten minutes or more. Practise every day until you are satisfied. Then move on to Step III: Regulate the Mind.)

Step III: Regulate the Mind

To regulate the mind, we use *mind-will (意念)*—a mental activity—to concentrate on a fixed spot or to direct the breath to a specific point in the body. *Mind-will (意念)* is generally used to discard distracting, disturbing thoughts and to stabilise our emotions so that we can enter into a state of calm and restfulness for the *qi* to be awakened.

Method: Training Mind Concentration

1. Exhale and inhale naturally through the nose. Keep calm and relaxed. Ignore all distractions. Concentrate on listening to something pleasant and rhythmic, such as the calling of birds, the chirping of insects, or the flow of water. Pay attention to the object, not the breathing. (Stay this way for 5 minutes.)

2. Concentrate exhaling and inhaling at the lower abdomen to train and nurture a "miniature

circuit" (小小周天)—a three-in-one (三向合一) movement to awaken the *qi* at the dantian elixir field (one and a half inches in from the navel).

3. Use *mind-will (意念)* to concentrate breathing lightly five times each at the navel, then at *ming-men* (命门), an energy point located opposite the navel at the back on the spine between the kidneys, and finally at *hui-yin* (会阴), an energy point at the lower part of the trunk between the anus and the genitals.

Figure 4: The Miniature Circuit Energy Points

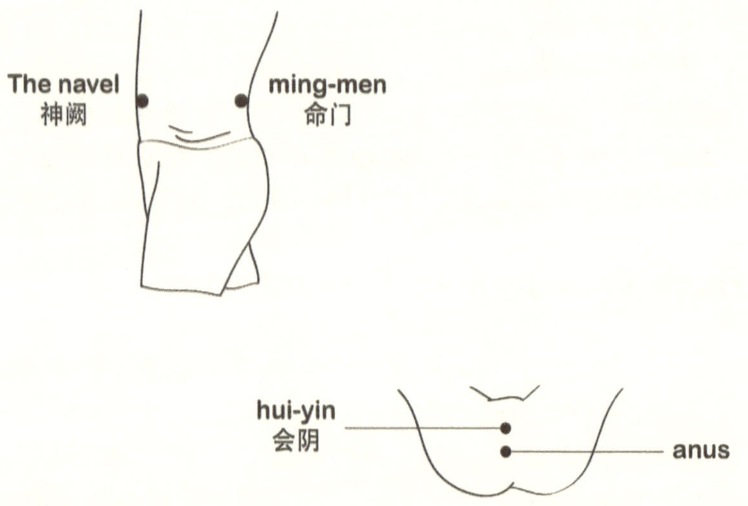

4. Use soft *mind-will (意念)* to follow an inverted triangular circuit.

   4.1 Inhale at the navel, follow the breath across the inside of the abdomen to the *ming-men* (命门) energy point. Exhale at *ming-men* down to the *hui-yin* (会阴) energy point. Then inhale at *hui-yin* up to the navel.

4.2 Now do the reverse. Exhale at the navel down to the *hui-yin* (会阴) energy point. Inhale at the *hui-yin* up to the *ming-men* (命门) energy point. Exhale at the *ming-men* across the abdomen to the navel.

Repeat this exercise at least 5 times with soft concentration.

Figure 5: The Inverted Triangular Circuit

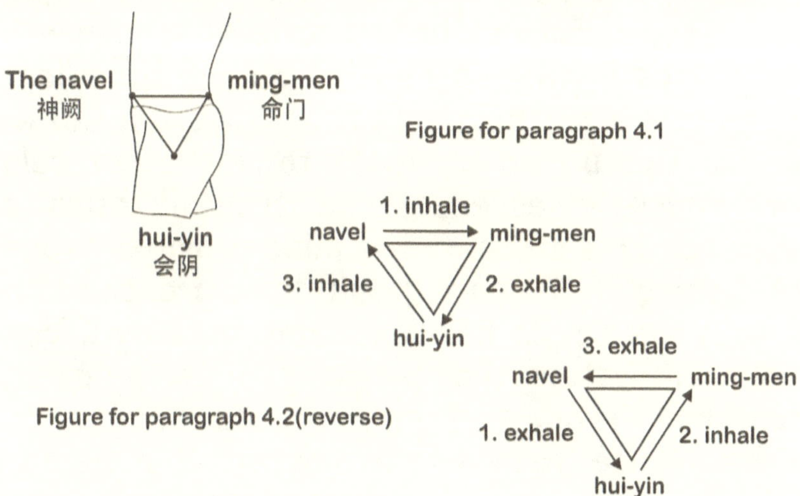

(Note: Pay attention to the point, not the breathing. Slowly let the concentration become faint, natural, and relaxed. Because the mind is not being used forcefully, we gradually move into a stage of calmness and restfulness. Various sensations will be felt. Different people experience different sensations. Some feel a tingling or warming effect, while others may feel cold and pain. Never compare your sensations with others. When you feel discomfort at any one point or tired of the concentration, stop the exercise and start again the next day.)

THE THREE-PHASE APPROACH TO MEDITATION: FROM HEALTHCARE TO ONENESS

The positive effects of healthcare through meditation are built up gradually. If we practise regularly and patiently, we will become better at it. If you follow the prescribed sequence of the phases in this approach, you will be able to experience a soothing effect on the brain and the nerves. This ultimately leads to relaxation, calm, restfulness, quiescence, and tranquilization of the mind. This state of the mind provides proper functioning of the parasympathetic branch of the nervous system. It has been confirmed by Qigong research masters that proper functioning of the parasympathetic system improves healing and health. Hence, to make the most of what we have to learn, we must avoid erratic practice. It is of the utmost importance to keep to learning each step in the manner laid down. Only then can we help ourselves to treat chronic health problems when they arise or prevent them from getting worse. Even when we have no problems, we can maintain good health to avoid having problems in the future.

Each phase has its own progressive steps so that we can pursue our development in stages. These steps allow us to reap positive results from our learning in accordance with individual needs.

PHASE I: STARTERS

The Phase I exercises lay the foundation for mental calmness and whole body relaxation. They create an opening for us to move smoothly into strengthening and invigorating the internal *qi* in Phase II.

Step One: Calm the Mind

1. Knock the upper teeth onto the lower teeth (first the molars, then the incisors and canines, each 9-18 times).

2. Use tip of the tongue to massage the upper and lower gums (first clockwise, then counter-clockwise, nine turns each).

3. Use the tip of the tongue to massage the hard palates (first clockwise, then counter-clockwise, nine turns each).

4. Swallow the saliva in three gulps, visualizing it going down to the lower abdomen dantian elixir field.

(Note: This whole exercise may be practised three times before moving in on Step Two.)

Step Two: Whole Body Relaxation

The Triple-Path Relaxation Exercise

This exercise requires us to use '*mind-will (意念)*' to direct our breathing slowly and lightly step by step down three distinctive paths to relieve tensions in the body and limbs. It has the effect of calming the mind and relaxing the whole body, which contributes to soothing the nerves to stabilize our emotions. Practise well; this exercise serves as a prelude for the brain to move more quickly into a restful state. After completing the three paths, we can move on to sitting silent for as long as we wish. If we can sit for thirty minutes each day, it will become a healthcare meditation nurturing the inherent *yuan qi* (元气) to become the vital life energy *zhen qi* (真气) (commonly referred to as *qi*) for health growth.

Figure 6: The Triple Paths

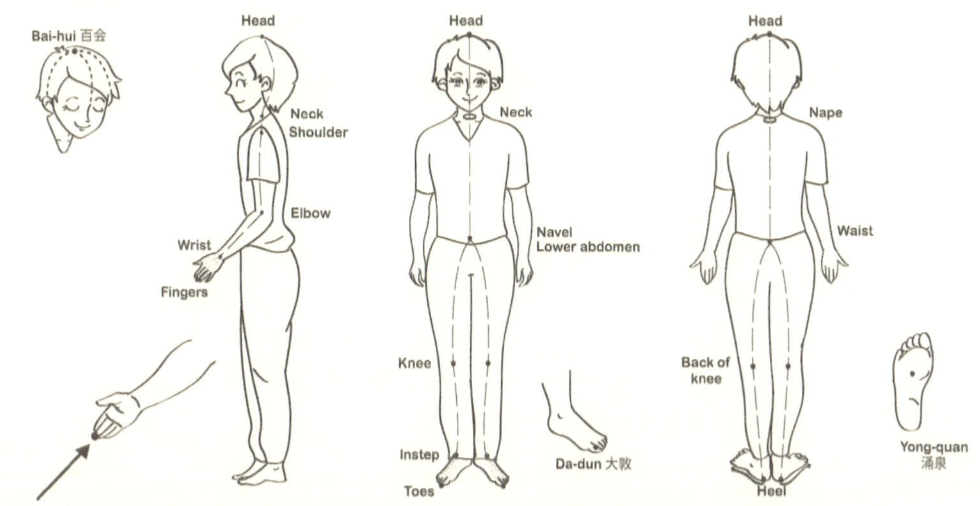

1. The Side Path

Head—neck—shoulders—elbows (respire 2x)—wrists—fingers. Concentrate and respire ten times at *zhong-chong* (中冲), the energy points at tips of middle fingers.

2. The Front Path

Head—neck—lower abdomen—knees (respire 2x)—instep—toes. Concentrate and respire ten times at the *da-dun* (大敦), the energy points on the big toes.

3. The Back Path

Head—nape—waist—back of knees (respire 2x)—heels—sole to toes. Concentrate and respire ten times at the *yong-quan (涌泉)*, the energy points on the soles.

Method:

1. Relax the First Path, then the Second Path, and finally the Third Path.

2. Inhale and exhale through the nose slowly and gently. Always begin inhaling at the head, and then exhale the breath down to the next specified location.

3. When inhaling, focus at the specified location. Exhale when moving down the path to the next location. Upon exhaling think of the word *soong (松)* which means "relax".

(Notes:

- During the practice, if you are feeling uncomfortable with lots of distracted thoughts and are not able to concentrate, or if you are not feeling relaxed, do not continue. Stop the practice. Take a walk to relax. Refer to Section Two (page 89-90) for the different walking exercises you can choose to do. Return to the practice again the next day.

- During the exercise, if your physical condition is hot, move more quickly down the path. On the contrary, if your physical condition is cold, breathe slowly and linger at each stop-point a little longer.

- During the exercise, when there is tension pain in a particular part of the body, relieve the pain by concentrating on the affected location. Then inhale through the nose and exhale through the mouth with slightly opened lips. During exhalation, blow out the word *soong (松)* meaning "relax" onto the affected part. Do this 9-18 times every day.

- At any time if you are having shortness of breath, stop the exercise. Inhale through the nose. Exhale through the mouth saying *hu (呼)* and use '*mind-will (意念)*' to follow the *qi* down to the navel. Do this 3-6 times and return to normal practice.

- Breathe at moderate speed. Exhaling or inhaling too fast and too forcefully triggers headaches; too slow or too light breathing causes sleepiness.

- If there are sensations of warmth, tingling, or quivering of muscles in some parts of the body when doing the exercise, do not interrupt the exercise. These are all normal reactions, indicating the *qi* is moving.

- If you are feeling good—comfortable, *physically relaxed, and mentally* rested—continue sitting with your eyes slightly closed. Breathe gently and naturally without the use of '*mind-will (意念)*.' Allow the mind to sink into a quiet state for thirty or more minutes of meditation. This is to enable the inherent *yuan qi* (元气) to transmute into a vital life energy *zhen qi* (真气) (commonly referred as *qi*). The longer we meditate, the better the chance for the *qi* to move out of the dantian and flow into and circulate the energy channels.

- When ready to stop, do the Winding Up exercise. The ascending, descending, opening, and closing movements return *qi* to its root (引气归元) at the lower abdomen *dantian (丹田)* elixir field to be stored.)

The "Winding Up" Exercise (引气归元)

Whenever we wish to close a meditation practice, we return *qi* to its root (引气归元) in the lower abdomen by doing the "Winding Up Exercise."

Method:

Inhale through the nose. Exhale through the mouth.

1. **Move the hands up and down three times.**

   Turn the hands with palms facing upwards and fingers facing each other. Inhale while slowly lifting hands upwards to mid-chest.

Then turn the palms downwards. Exhale while slowly returning hands to the lower abdomen.

2. **Move the hands sideways three times.**

At the lower abdomen, turn the hands with back of palms facing each other, fingers hanging down. Inhale while slowly pushing the hands apart to the sides of the abdomen.

Then turn the palms inward. Exhale while bringing hands back towards the navel, directing the qi into the dantian.

3. **Massage the abdomen.**

Place one palm over the other on the navel. Breathe naturally and focus on the navel while rubbing in clockwise and counter-clockwise motion (9-18 times each.) When rubbing, avoid exerting strength so that the hands are not stiff and rigid. Rubbing should be natural, gentle, and continuous. If there is a soft sensation in the abdomen, it is normal.

4. **Nurture the dantian elixir field.**

With palms remaining cupped over the navel, nurture the dantian (静养丹田) by letting go of all concentration, and breathe naturally for at least two minutes.

5. Massage the face.

Warm the hands by rubbing the palms together twelve times. Push the hands lightly up and down the face 9-18 times or as you wish.

6. Stand up slowly.

Either lightly stamp the feet on the ground fifty or a hundred times or take a slow walk for at least five minutes.

(Note: The next day, if you are feeling at ease and comfortable, move in on Phase II. If not, carry on with doing the Triple Path exercise for as long as you need to until you are ready to move on.)

PHASE II: DIRECTING QI FLOW INTO THE SMALL AND LARGE HEAVENLY CIRCUIT

Phase II involves two steps in training and nurturing the internal *qi* to flow out of the lower abdominal dantian elixir field and circulate into the *qi* channels (经络). These steps are progressively designed, starting from *training* the mind to concentrate on getting rid of distracting thoughts to *nurturing* the mind into mental calm and restfulness. When the *qi* circulates the *ren-du* midline channels in a Small Heavenly Circuit, the nurturing exercise enhances the mind to move slowly into a state of quiescence to enable the *qi* to automatically self-circulate into a Large Heavenly Circuit and eventually covering all *qi* channels (经络) lining the body.

Figure 7: Small and Large Heavenly Circuits

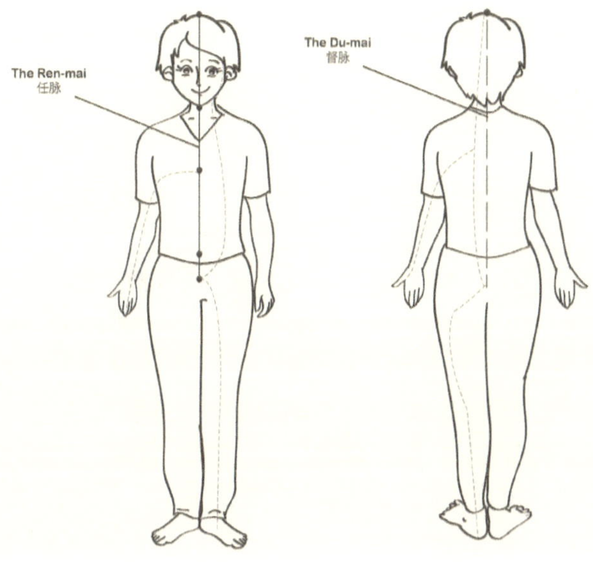

What Is Training and Nurturing?

Training and nurturing complement each other in helping us develop a breath that is slow, smooth, long, and deep, and a mind that is calm, restful, and finally quiescent. At the restful stage, nurturing silently allows the breath to build up the *qi* to move out of the lower abdominal dantian elixir field into the *ren-du* midline channels. Then with training and nurturing at the *ren-du mai* (任督脉) midline channels, this *qi* circulates in a Small Heavenly Circuit until the mind reaches a quiescent stage, and the *qi* becomes a potent force to move automatically into the Large Heavenly Circuit, where it eventually covers all *qi* channels in the body for health maximisation.

Step I: Train and Nurture *Qi* at Lower Dantian Elixir Field

Method

1. **"Training Stage."** Sit in silence. Start by breathing slowly and gently into the navel for five to ten minutes. Then use 'mind-will 意念' to listen to the breathing and sense the rise-and-fall movement of the lower abdomen. Do not exert *'mind-will (意念)'* to upset the gentle breathing and the rise-and-fall movement of the abdomen. This exercise, besides training the mind to concentrate on getting rid of distracting thoughts by listening and sensing movements in the lower abdomen, also lays the foundation for us to be able to listen and sense changes in our body as signals to oncoming diseases in future years.

   Do five cycles of exhalation-inhalation gently listening to the breath, and softly sensing the abdominal movement. Then move on to the nurturing stage.

   (Note: If we are a weak and nervous person, alternate concentration between navel and the *ming-men* energy point.)

2. "**Nurturing Stage.**" Continuing from above, we remain sitting in silence and breathing gently and softly into the lower abdomen. We slowly weaken our '*mind-will (意念)*' to allow the listening of the breath and sensing of the abdominal movement to fade out. In this way, we free our mind of thinking so as to be able to nurture the breath and the *qi*. The whole exercise gradually becomes natural and relaxed, allowing the breathing to become slow, smooth, long, and deep, and the mind gradually sinks into a stage of calm, restfulness, and finally quiescence. There are times when a warming, tingling, or quivering sensation is felt in some parts of the body. Such a sensation indicates the internal energy *qi* is moving.

   (Note: At this moment most of us tend to be distracted, and we try to use '*mind-will (意念)*' to direct the breathing to pursue more sensations. Never do things that would cause your mind to be in an excitable or stressful state. Sensations are normal reactions. Do not think about them. Thinking interferes with movement of the *qi*.)

   Remain sitting silently as long as you are feeling relaxed and comfortable. The moment stray thoughts stream into the mind, return to do five cycles of training at the lower abdomen, and then return to the nurturing again.

(Note: Training and nurturing complement each other. This is the way to rid our mind of distracting thoughts, to replenish the *qi* that is lost during the exercise, and to strengthen the existing *qi* to flow and circulate freely.)

Do this exercise for at least twenty minutes. Close the practice by returning all *qi* to its root (引气归元) in the lower abdomen by doing the Winding Up exercise (page 20-22).

The next day, if not feeling at ease and comfortable to move in on Step II, repeat Step I exercise for another day or many more days until ready to move on.

Step II: Train and Nurture Qi at the Ren-Du Mai (任督脉) Midline Channels in a Small Heavenly Circuit;

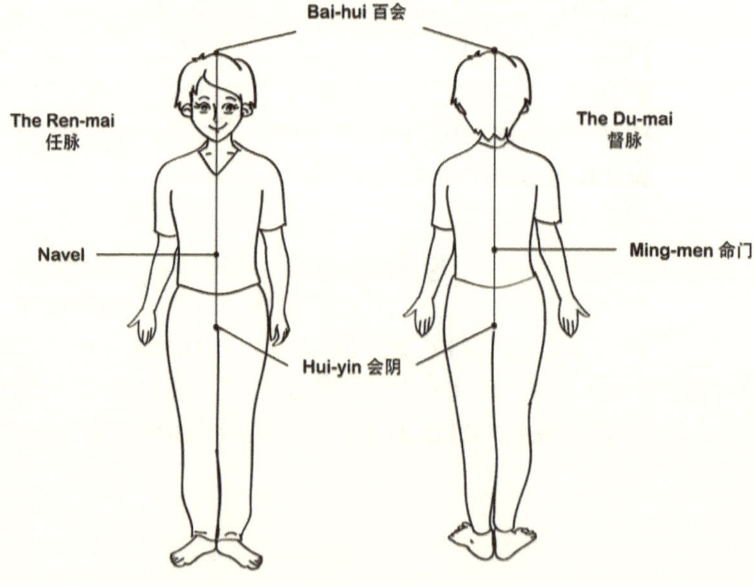

Method:

1. **"Training Stage."** Sit in silence. Start by breathing slowly and gently into the navel for at least five minutes. Then use 'mind-will 意念' to direct the *qi* flow and circulation.

    i. Inhale into the navel, then exhale with '*mind-will (意念)*' following the *qi* down to the *hui-yin* (会阴).

    ii. Inhale into the *hui-yin* (会阴). Use '*mind-will(意念)*' to follow the inhalation up the spine to the *ming-men* (命门), and then exhale.

    iii. Inhale into the *ming-men* (命门). Use '*mind-will (意念)*' to follow the inhalation up the spine to the *bai-hui* (百会) energy point at the top of the head. Exhale into the *bai-hui* (百会). Stop at this point to inhale-exhale a few times or more until there is a feeling of warm power in the forehead and face. Ignore the sensation and carry on with the next step.

    iv. Inhale at the *bai-hui* (百会), and then exhale with '*mind-will (意念)*' following the exhalation down to the navel at the lower abdomen (the action of sinking *qi* down to the dantian (气沉丹田).

This completes circulation of *qi* into the Small Heavenly Circuit.

Repeat the whole exercise 3-5 times. Gradually let go of the conscious concentration that uses '*mind-will (意念)*' to direct the flow and circulation of *qi* and allow our meditation to move into the nurturing stage.

2. **"Nurturing Stage."** Continuing from above, remain sitting in silence and focus your breathing gently and softly at the navel for five to ten minutes. Slowly weaken the '*mind-will (意念)*' and let the concentration fade out. In this way we free our mind of thinking so as to be able to nurture the breath and the *qi*. Remain sitting silently for as long as you are feeling relaxed and comfortable. Without the need to concentrate, the breathing becomes slow, smooth, long, and deep, and the mind gradually sinks from a state of calm and restfulness into one of quiescence. There are times when a warming, tingling, or quivering sensation is felt at some parts of the body. Such a sensation indicates the internal energy *qi* is flowing and circulating.

(Note: At this moment, most of us tend to be distracted and try to use '*mind-will (意念)*' to direct the breathing to pursue more sensations. Never do things that would cause your mind to be in an excitable or stressful state. Sensations are normal reactions. Do not think about them. Thinking interferes with movement of the *qi*. The moment stray thoughts stream into the mind, return to do 5 times of training at the *ren-du mai* (任督脉) midline channels as described above in the Training Stage. Then return to nurturing.)

It has been said by my meditation Master, Ma Ji Ren, a veteran Qigong practitioner, that as the *qi* flows and circulates up and down the *ren-du* midline channels in a Small Heavenly Circuit, the yin-yang energy harmonises. There is no excess or deficiency of one over the other to upset the flow or cause sickness. Instead, the balance enables the *qi* to gather more power and build up a warm current to clear all clogs and blocks along the circuit (especially the chakras.) In this way the potent *qi* begins to strengthen its smooth flow and circulates more vigorously through the circuit; then it gradually self-circulates into a Large Heavenly Circuit and eventually into all other channels lining the body.

(Note: The *ren* mai (任脉) in the front of the body has yin energy. The *du* mai (督脉) at the back of the body along the spine carries yang energy. When *qi* flows and circulates within these two midline channels in a circuit, the yin-yang energy *qi* eventually harmonises. After a few circulations, there is no more excess or deficiency of one over the other to cause upsets in the flow of *qi* and sickness. There are twenty-four energy points along the *ren* mai (任脉) and twenty-eight energy points along the *du mai* (督脉). When our nourished *qi* flows along these energy points and the nutrient-carrying blood cells flow through the blood streams, together they spur healing effects on the internal organs and nervous system to better our health and increase our life expectancy.

Qi Reactions in the Large Heavenly Circuit

When we remain sitting calmly, restfully, and quiescently, flow and circulation of the *qi* will continue. However, there are times when we are disturbed by external environmental distractions or some peculiar internal sensations, and then stray thoughts seep into the mind.

To get rid of them, look inwardly into the lower abdominal dantian, and listen to the steady rhythm of the breath. After five cycles of exhalation-inhalation, slowly fade out the inward looking and listening and do nurturing of the *qi* with slow and gentle breathing. Little by little a warm and comfortable sensation is felt in the lower abdomen and at the side of the abdomen below the rib cage or in the fingers and toes. This indicates that the strengthened and invigorated *qi* has moved into the channels.

Continue the nurturing. With a balanced yin-yang energy and no more blockages along the *ren-du* (任督脉) midline channels, our strong *qi* automatically flows and circulates into a Large Heavenly Circuit

(大周天), opening up all the *qi* channels (*jing-luo* (经络)) that line all parts of the body. A warm tingling sensation can be felt in the arms, hands, and legs. Ignore this and continue from here, our healthcare meditation, for as long as we wish.

This stage makes possible the body's final transmutation of the "three treasures" that constitute human life—the *jing (精)* essence fluid, *qi* (气) energy force, and *shen* (神) spiritual consciousness. *Jing (精)*, the foundation for life, is primarily stored in the kidneys and the sexual organs. *Qi* (气), the root of life, is the energy force behind the functional activities of our body system. *Shen* (神), the spiritual consciousness, is the manifestation of all our mental and physical activities and functions of the five senses and thoughts. Together with blood, *jing-qi-shen* (精气神) are the basic life substances in our body that sustain healthy functions of the internal organs and the whole body system.

With *jing-qi-shen* (精气神) in harmony, along with the smooth circulation of the powerful *qi*, the nutrient-carrying blood is influenced to circulate into the blood streams of the visceral organs. Research studies and clinical experiments have confirmed that *qi* and blood have a soothing and regulating effect on the brain and nerves. They also nurture and strengthen the functions of the central nervous system, the circulatory system, and the respiratory, digestive, lymphatic and endocrine systems. They also improve the immune system to maintain good health and longevity. This powerful *qi* is indeed the vital life-healing energy that has a strong influence on healthcare. We help ourselves to treat chronic health problems when they arise or prevent them from getting worse. Even when we have no problems, we maintain good health to avoid having problems in the future.

The central belief in Traditional Chinese Qigong practice is that as *qi* circulates with yin-yang energy in balance and with no blockages along the *qi* channels, more and more *qi* amasses, and more and more power gathers. This potent, enriched, and strengthened *qi*, when circulating in the Large Heavenly Circuit, induces better flow and circulation of blood cells into the blood streams and thus into all the internal organs and body systems. This logic is the same as what has been observed by Chinese physicians—that *qi* is essentially the leader of blood. If *qi* is weak, blood circulation will be enfeebled and sickness will befall on us. Hence, in both traditional Chinese medicine and Qigong practices, if *qi* in our body flows and circulates smoothly around both the Small and Large Heavenly Circuits, we are less likely to fall sick.

(Note: In each day of our meditation, if we have no wish to move in on the next step or phase, we may close the practice by doing the Winding Up exercise described on page 20-22 to return all *qi* to its root (引气归元) in the lower abdomen. Do the Phase II exercise every day for up to two years or more, as you wish, before moving on to Phase III for oneness meditation. When the day comes that you are feeling calm and restful and are sensing fitness, instead of winding up the exercise, carry on with the quiescent sitting and move into oneness meditation. In such an instance, we are continuing the meditation for as long as sixty minutes.

PHASE III: ONENESS MEDITATION

Phase Three leads us into perfect stillness of mind in a state of "nothingness" to attain tranquillity. The exercises in this phase make possible the achievement of two ultimate aims in meditation practice. The first is final transmutation into a spiritual component in its purest form of the three "treasures" of human life—the essence fluid *jing* 精, the energy force *qi* 气, and the spiritual consciousness *shen* (神). These three components of *jing (精)—qi* (气)*—shen* (神)—the basic life substances in our body—interplay with one another to sustain healthy functions of the whole body system. The second aim is the awakening of the spirit to achieve "oneness" (union) with the laws of nature. Such can only be achieved through our oneness meditation.

Oneness meditation is an advanced stage in meditation. It has in it an essence of spirituality—the ending of all earthly thoughts to move into a different dimension of the ultimate reality that is beyond time and space. Oneness enables us to attain transcendental bliss; it unfolds our latent creative intelligence to maintain an intelligence that is creatively perceptive with acumen for good judgment; and it evokes the innate humane nature that is personified in our character and personality.

The significant value of this form of meditation is the removal of all mental confusion so that our creative intelligence can surface. Creative intelligence is the wisdom providing clear perception and insight into every thought and action in our daily encounters with life.

For oneness meditation, we can either start right away after completing Phase II or we can embark on doing Phase III alone. In this case, the following method is to be used.

Method

Step 1: Quiescence into Tranquillity

1. Try to choose an environment that is quiet and free from noise and other distractions. Sit in silence. Start with sinking the word *kong* (空) into the lower abdomen. Inhale through the nose, thinking of the word *kong* (空). Exhale slowly and gently using '*mind-will (意念)*' to sink the word *kong* (空) into the lower abdomen. During the exercise, listen to the word *kong* (空) sinking into the lower abdomen. This exercise allows the mind to concentrate so that it can get rid of distracting thoughts.

Repeat the inhalation-exhalation five to nine times at the navel.

2. Fade out the listening. Instead, sense the rise-and-fall movement of the lower abdomen. Do not exert *'mind-will (意念)'* to upset the gentle breathing and the rise-and-fall movement of the abdomen. Slowly let go of all listening and sensing. Continue breathing gently at the lower abdomen, calmly and restfully.

3. Nurture the *qi* by sitting in silence, letting go of all concentration and remaining calm and restful. We may feel other peculiar sensations. Sensations are normal reactions that indicate the internal energy *qi* is moving. Do not think about them. Thinking interferes with movement of the *qi*. By not thinking, we free our mind to nurture the breath and the *qi*. We allow the *qi* at the dantian elixir field to accrue and strengthen by itself. The time comes when a current of warm *qi* is naturally felt at different parts of the body. This indicates that *qi* is circulating. Whenever stray thoughts stream into the mind, return to conscious breathing into the navel while thinking of the word *kong* (空). Do five to nine cycles of inhalation-exhalation. Gradually return to the nurturing stage of meditation.

4. The whole meditation exercise gradually becomes natural and relaxed, allowing the

breathing to become slow, smooth, long, and deep, and the mind gradually sinks into a stage of quiescence, able to ignore all environmental noise and colour. Remain sitting in quiescence. The steady rhythm of the slow, smooth, long, and deep breathing will eventually become subtle and soft—almost imperceptible. Continue sitting for at least forty-five minutes to an hour.

Let the subtle and soft breath go on with no exertion of '*mind-will (意念)*'. Allow the mind to move gradually from quiescence into tranquillity. Let it be totally empty of thoughts, drifting into a deep level of nothingness, reposing in the true nature of ultimate reality, and attaining a harmonious, mystical union of oneness with nature's law. This moment of silent nothingness brings forth transcendental bliss, leaving inside us a deep feeling of ease and calmness and a deep sense of inner renewal. This is our ultimate achievement in oneness meditation.

From my experience with oneness meditation, silent nothingness brought forth transcendental bliss, but the blissfulness could not last long—only a minute or so—before the mind became conscious of the immediate surroundings again. Yet this short moment of silent nothingness left a deep feeling of ease and calmness and a deep sense of inner renewal. After a few years of constant and disciplined practice, a satisfying outcome is when my thoughts and actions are tied in with an insight into seeing the true nature of things around me with the finest aspect of clear thinking and clear perception.

(Note: It may take years to arrive at this stage of meditation. All depends on the individual's physical condition and lifestyle. It takes months, sometimes years, to achieve satisfaction and comfort for this stage of meditation, especially for those of us who are not in good health but have the desire to plunge into oneness meditation without going through the stages of healthcare in Phases I and II. If we do progress to Phase III from Phase II, we have the following advantages:

1. We have the benefit of Phase II qi circulation strength to circulate in a systematic order round the body in the gentlest and most effective way.

2. We have the advantage of a quiescent mind to help in accelerating tranquillity, to help our breathing to become subtle and soft—almost imperceptible—leading to final achievement of the mind drifting into a deep level of nothingness.

3. We have the advantage of inheriting the life healing qi that has been strengthened and powered during its flow and circulation in the Large Heavenly Circuit and in all other qi channels.)

MATTERS OF SIGNIFICANT IMPORTANCE

1. The main purpose of healthcare meditation is to cultivate and nurture the inherent yuan qi元气 to become a vital life energy *zhen qi* (真气) (commonly referred as *qi*) for healing damaged cells and to maintain good health.

2. Meditate in a pleasant environment where you can breathe in fresh air at sunrise. Engage in thirty or forty-five minutes to an hour of meditation, if not daily, at least three times a week.

3. Breathing should always be natural, gentle at the beginning, eventually allowing the breath to become slow, smooth, long, and deep, and finally soft and subtle. Do not inhale fully—eighty or ninety per cent is enough—and do not exhale forcefully.

4. Remember that meditation requires constant practice and discipline. Meditation is the gentlest and most effective way of nurturing the *qi* for physical, mental, and spiritual health. "Perseverance is the secret of success."

5. The approach to healthcare meditation in Phases I and II can be used by any of us when recovering from illness, healing from an injury, or undergoing fatigue or sleeplessness.

6. Do each step in each phase repeatedly until you feel calm, restfully relaxed, comfortable, and satisfied.

7. If we find we have the knack of attaining quiescence and *qi* circulation in an instant, we can start straight off on Phase II or III.

8. If at any moment our lifestyle should change and bring on tension and stress, we should choose to do the basic exercises to regulate the breathing and the mind, gradually move on to Phase I to calm the mind and relax the whole body.

9. To make the most of what we have to learn and to avoid erratic practice, it is of the utmost importance to keep to learning each step in the manner laid down.

10. Do not be impatient with distracting thoughts. To get rid of them, concentrate on the training part of the exercise. Should these distracting thoughts linger on, open your eyes and massage your head with both hands. Then massage the inner side of the wrist (two centimetres away

from the transverse wrinkles.) Then return to the exercise.

11. If you experience sensations of warmth, cold, slight pain, tingling of muscles, and slight quivering at the tips of fingers or toes or in the arms and legs during exercise, do not interrupt, as these are normal reactions.

12. Do not seek to have such sensations. They surface according to our physical conditions. Sensations of warmth in one part of the body and cold in another part are indications of yin-yang energy imbalance or clogs at the channels. Just continue with the exercise until the yin-yang energy is in balance and lends its force to the *qi* to clear the blocks and clogs in the channels.

13. Our lifestyle, the type of food we eat, and the amount of fresh air we breathe in can influence our capacity to benefit fully from my form of healthcare and oneness meditation. For this reason, we need to regulate our work schedule, avoid erratic sleeping hours, and eliminate all unhealthy habits.

14. We should scale our food consumption with advice from a dietician combined with some general nutritional supplementation as advised by the doctor.

15. Those of us who are beginners must never allow the slow pace and sense of isolation that is often

experienced in meditation to deter us from success. We must discipline ourselves to reset our daily schedule and our sleeping patterns and to create time for exposure to fresh air and sunshine. Do not rush through all the exercises.

16. Those who already have prior knowledge of meditation and have no health problems may go straight into Phase III to attain their oneness with nature.

17. If you experience dizziness, feeling cold, or shivering, check on your breathing. Try not to hold the breath at any one point too long. Also, check whether your '*mind-will (意念)*' or breathing is overly forceful. Check whether your posture is relaxed—not stiff and rigid.

    (Note: If such reactions continue or if they are accompanied by faintness, nausea, severe shortness of breath, cold or profuse sweating all over the body during practice, violent shaking, extreme discomfort, or severe pain, stop the meditation. Do a *qi* regulation exercise or a free walking exercise (Section II, page 86-90). If such severe reactions persist more than three times in succession, consult a doctor. When you decide to resume practice, do the Phase I meditation again and again until you feel at ease and comfortable.)

18. Good posture, the exercises on breathing and on calming the mind, and the triple-path

relaxation provide mental and physical relaxation. The exercise on training and nurturing the *qi* with slow, smooth, long, and deep breathing builds up and strengthens the *qi* in the dantian elixir field. The end result much depends on our discipline in practice and our mental, physical, and emotional condition at the time of practice.

DOS AND DON'TS IN MEDITATION

The Dos

- Always take your first lesson on meditation from an experienced person.
- Keep to one form of meditation.
- Sit facing the magnetic field—either north or south.
- Exercise in an area that is well ventilated.
- Keep the mind in a cheerful frame during exercise. Put on a smile.
- Empty your bladder before starting on the exercise.
- Put on loose-fitting clothes.
- Eat warm food and take a warm drink.

- Swallow your saliva if it comes on.
- Meditate in a bright, fresh and pleasant environment.

The Don'ts

- Do not embark on different styles of meditation from different school of thoughts at one time.
- For women, do not meditate during menstruation. You may do the natural breathing exercise.
- Do not meditate in darkness or with a bright light shining on the face.
- Do not sit facing the sun.
- Do not meditate when there is thunder and lightning or during an eclipse of the sun or the moon.
- Do not put on air-conditioning or fans. Avoid direct draught to keep from catching the wind and cold.
- Do not continue to meditate if you find the surroundings distracting or the noise getting on your nerves.

- Do not endure tightness around the chest, waist, wrists, fingers, knees, or toes.
- Do not meditate when feeling depressed.
- If you are a beginner, do not meditate when travelling in a car, bus, ship, or plane.
- Do not meditate immediately after a full meal, and do not meditate when hungry.
- Do not meditate if your body temperature exceeds 38°C. Do consult a doctor.
- Do not smoke thirty minutes before or after the practice. (Eventually smokers will be able to stop smoking.)
- Do not eat, drink, or wash immediately after meditation.
- Do not take alcoholic drinks immediately before or after meditation.
- Do not get involved in things that would cause you anxieties immediately before or after meditation.
- Do not embark on self-aid when you encounter abnormalities during and after meditation. Always consult the doctor first.

Section Two

Mobile Qigong

(*Da Yan Liu Zi Gong* 大雁六字功)

A '*Qi*' Energy Harmonising Exercise
with Fluid Movements, Mind-will, and a Breathing
Discipline to Regulate Healthy Functions
of the Body's Visceral Organs, Lymphatic,
And Endocrine Systems

UNDERSTANDING *DA YAN LIU ZI GONG* (大雁六字功)

The ancient Chinese discovered that breathing exercises promote the circulation of *qi* and blood, while physical movements improve functions of the joints, ligaments, and muscles. Based on these beliefs, *da yan liu zi gong* 大雁六字功 was founded by my Qigong Master Shen He Nian. It comprises seven therapeutic exercise regimens. 'Mind-will意念', breathing disciplines, and physical movements are integral part of the exercises to awaken and nurture the life healing energy *zhen qi* (真气) to flow into the body organs and systems to repair cells to self-heal chronic ailments.

DISTINGUISHING FEATURES

Da yan liu zi gong (大雁六字功) has an exact role to play in the processing, storage, and distribution of *qi* to the organs and systems to strengthen each of its functions so as to restore and maintain good health. It has four distinguished features:

1. **Adopt actions of the bean goose.** Four of the seven exercise regimens in *da yan liu zi gong* (大雁六字功) imitate actions of the bean goose. The principal exercise regimen that harmonizes the yin-yang energy imitates the take-off and landing (大雁起落) action. The liver exercise regimen imitates the action of spreading out and folding of wings from front to back (前后展翅). The lung exercise regimen imitates the action on dipping of wings to splash water onto the body (大雁拍水). And the triple-heater exercise regimen imitates the action of looking left and right before taking flight (左右看足). These four actions of the bean goose, together with the smooth and flowing grace of the other three movements that include the heart (抱颈颠顶), the spleen (托天动地), and the kidneys (左顾右盼), exude calmness and serenity. These factors create a feeling of general ease and comfortable relaxation—an essential step to good health.

2. **Embrace a six-character formula** (六字诀). *Da yan liu zi gong* (大雁六字功) embraces a six-character formula (六字诀) as a

technique to clear adverse energies (邪气) present in the body organs and systems. Adverse energies are generally caused by environmental factors that trigger our physical constitution to be hot, cold, dry, or damp, causing a deficiency or an excess in our yin-yang energy system. The six characters are *xu (嘘)* (pronounce as "she") for the liver, *ke (呵)* (pronounce as "ker") for the heart, *hu (呼)* (pronounce as "hoo") for the spleen, *si (四)* for the lungs, *chui (吹)* for the kidneys, and *xi (嘻)* (pronounce as "see") for the triple-heater encompassing the lymphatic and endocrine systems. The technique involves co-ordinating the reading of the word in the mind with movement of the limbs during one of the exhalation processes. After exhaling, we inhale the breath to nurture the liver (养肝), nourish the heart (补心), invigorate the spleen (健脾), moisturize the lungs (润肺), strengthen the kidneys (强肾), regulate the triple-heater (理三焦), sequentially, the lymphatic and endocrine systems.

3. **An all-inclusive set of six positions.** Da yan liu zi gong 大雁六字功 has an all-inclusive set of six positions in which the waist is used as the central pivot, balancing the trunk to turn left and then right, bend forward and then backward, move upward and then downward. The flowing, smooth, graceful, elegant movements outwardly look fluid, but they possess an internal strength to strengthen

the spine and improve the functions of the joints, ligaments, and muscles. The change in positions that involves movement of arms and legs, improves *qi* and blood circulation to the entire body up to the extremities of fingers and toes.

4. **Easy to learn.** *Da yan liu zi gong* (大雁六字功) is easy to learn. The mobile movements are safe for practice by young and old, sick and healthy, as they require only moderate physical exertion. The posture is elegant, and the movements in each exercise regimen are quite simple. It can be practised at any convenient time and within a one square metre of space, indoors or outdoors. We may practise either the complete set of seven exercise regimens at one go or a particular regimen repeatedly to help to relieve a particular ailment.

ROLE IN HEALTHCARE

Da yan liu zi gong (大雁六字功) involves seven individual exercise regimens with a combination of '*mind-will (意念)*', symmetrical movements, and a breathing discipline to restore the balance of *qi* in the body organs and systems to stimulate their self-healing efficacies. The principal regimen harmonises the yin-yang energy to balance excesses and deficiencies of chills and heat in the body system. Yin-yang equanimity acts as a force to activate the *qi* to circulate smoothly into the energy channels. The other six regimens direct *qi* and blood to flow smoothly into the visceral organs and triple-heater *qi* channels to strengthen their functional activities, providing resistance to diseases and thus maintaining good health.

Each exercise regimen is an integration of '*mind-will (意念)*' and breathing, breathing and physical movement. This involves deep concentration at the start of the exercise. When we arrive at the stage when the physical movements are integrated with the breathing exercises and we are using '*mind-will (意念)*' to concentrate on the movements of the hands and specific acupuncture points, mental disruptions and emotional irritations are eliminated. As the movements and breathing are symmetrical, the concentration gradually becomes soft and light. The body muscles relax and become tension-free, and the mind becomes unperturbed and restful, the breathing gentle and natural. Finally, the whole self enters a high degree of tranquillity, feeling the smooth flow of *qi* and blood round the body. This circulation supplies the needed nutrition and life-nourishing elements, not only to help ward off diseases associated with the body organs and systems, but also to improve the immune, brain, and central nerve functions.

Our health is constantly affected by seasonal and environmental changes. In Traditional Chinese Qigong (TCQ), wind, heat, coldness, dryness, or dampness are regarded as adverse *energies (邪气)*

that upset the equilibrium of the *qi* system in the body. This often leads to weakening of the *qi* flow in the energy channels. Such adverse conditions are likely to cause dysfunction of the body organs and body systems—the origin of diseases. Applying the six-character formula in our practice is most fitting for maximising good health.

From my own experience, after six months of constant practice at regular hours, I found my physical fitness and power of perception markedly improved and my emotions more stabilized—calm and composed, not easily unruffled. My grip strength has also been reinforced with improved flexibility. From this experience, I can safely say that if we practise *da yan liu zi gong* (大雁六字功) regularly, we will have less chance of getting seriously ill and more chance of getting healed.

THE PRACTICE

In *da yan liu zi gong* (大雁六字功) the external movements and the breathing disciplines are regulated by '*mind-will (意念)*'. We begin our lessons by first concentrating on the physical movements that are regulated by the mind. When these become natural and comfortable, we proceed to the next stage, which involves combining the physical movements with the breathing exercises.

During each practice, we need to relax the muscles and at the same time calm the mind and breathe naturally. To achieve results, each exercise regimen is repeated seven times. (Doing the exercise on the left and then the right is regarded as one count.) Each movement must be at an exact level with moderate speed and strength. Remember not to be stiff. In this way we keep our muscles as relaxed as possible to ensure smooth and graceful flow of movements. '*Mind-will (意念)*' is used softly to stimulate and direct the internal *qi* and blood to circulate into the body organs and systems.

Upon completion of all the regimens, stand in a meditative posture with the feet together or apart and the palms cupped over the navel. With eyes dropped to the ground, breathe gently and naturally into the lower abdomen. This closing posture keeps us physically relaxed and mentally calm for a while to allow the *qi* to move from the channels into the lower abdominal dantian to be stored.

REGULATING THE BODY

Traditional Chinese Qigong Masters held that if our posture is not correct while exercising, our breathing will be upset, our mind will be disturbed, our spirit will be distraughted, and—most undesirable—the flow of internal *qi* will be disrupted.

As *da yan liu zi gong* (大雁六字功) is a mobile exercise, the posture adopted throughout is the standing style. In standing, we keep the body upright to force the back muscles to contract in support of the spine. "Standing naturally as straight as a pine tree rooted to the earth" is to maintain a firm posture to ensure steadiness and strength.

Standing Posture (Hands Cupped)

(See figure 2, page 6 in Section I.)

This standing posture can be used for standing meditation. Stand with heels together and the front part of feet opened to one fist's width between the big toes. Place the weight of the body onto the soles of feet. Stand firmly like a rooted pine tree. Keep the head upright. Close the mouth gently. Tuck in the chin. Drop the shoulders slightly. Keep the nose in a straight line with the navel. Flex the knees. Flex the elbows, while placing both palms facing inwards one on top the other on the navel. Eyes either look horizontally straight ahead or you can lower the eyelids to look on the ground.

The Legs

Movement of the legs improves blood circulation to the toes.

1. **When standing feet apart.** Move the left foot to the width of the shoulders. Place the right foot squarely on the ground to support your body weight as the left foot is moved. As in the exercise regimen on "Spleen and

Stomach", the body is lowered to a semi-squat position.

2. **When standing with one leg ahead of the other**. Always move the left leg first, then the right leg. Move one leg forward one step at an acceptable distance. When required, move the forward leg forward, bent like a bow with the knee above the toes. The hind leg stays at the same spot with the foot firmly on the ground and with the hip supporting the body weight. Sometimes the forward leg rests the heel lightly on the ground with toes tilted upward, while the hind leg, with knee bent, stays with the foot firmly on the ground and the hip supporting the body weight (as in the "Liver" exercise regimen.)

Hands. The palm is slightly cupped in with fingers and thumb naturally extended in a curve. (Place the palm on top of the head to get the curve.) Movement of the hands is divided into parts, for example, pressing the palms downward, flexing the fingers, and rotating the fists. Flexing and letting go of the fingers improves blood circulation to the finger tips.

Fist. Place the thumb at the base of the ring finger. The other four fingers are folded and placed lightly over the thumb. Do not tense up the fingers.

Arms. Movement of the arms can consist of raising the arms to a horizontal level, raising them up further, pulling them back down to the original horizontal level, and then pressing them downward.

Waist. The waist is the main axis of the body. In all the exercise regimens, the waist acts as the pivot supporting the strength to exercise the spine. The waist is linked to the legs. The legs further strengthen the spine and increase the movement range of the body trunk. The trunk is moved in six directions—turned left and right, bent forward and backward, raised and lowered.

Head and Eyes. The head and eyes always follow the hand movements.

REGULATING THE BREATHING

In *da yan liu zi gong* (大雁六字功), the breathing must be slow, smooth, long, and deep. Gently inhale through the nose and exhale through the mouth. The air we inhale must be perfectly adequate for us not to be short of breath—not too much nor too little. When we come to the stage of getting rid of the adverse energies, use the six-character formula (六字诀). Say each specified word in the mind when exhaling the breath through the mouth.

The breathing is developed step by step. When practising, we try to coordinate our breathing with the physical movements of the arms. As beginners, we will first learn how to perform each movement in each exercise regimen correctly with natural and smooth breathing. When we feel we can perform the exercises comfortably—feeling relaxed with our mind calm and restful—we shall then begin to pay attention to the breathing disciplines with the use of '*mind-will (意念).*'

My Qigong Master emphasized the need to avoid abnormal breathing during the exercise. Abnormal breathing means purposefully holding the breath or taking short breaths. This form of breathing can be exhausting and may cause injury to the organs.

Regulating the Mind

The mind commands the functions of all the internal organs. So any stressful activities or minor emotional disturbances may affect the functions of these organs. A good way to be calm and relaxed before starting the exercise is to stand upright with hands cupped over the navel and then use '*mind-will (意念)*' to inhale from the nose and exhale down the chest into the lower abdomen. This releases tightness in the chest and head to sink the *qi* into the dantian (气沉丹田). Each time before you start the practice, do this for thirty seconds or up to two minutes so that when performing the exercises, the body, breathing, and mind gradually become one integrated whole.

During the exercise '*mind-will (意念)*' is used softly to direct our concentration to different parts of the body during movements of our hands, arms, and legs. We concentrate:

1. At the tips of the ten fingers and toes.

2. At energy points at the lower abdomen dantian, or at *shan-zhong* (膻中) on the chest, or at *lao-gong* (劳宫) on the palms, or at *yong-quan* (涌泉) at the sole of the feet.

3. In front of the body.

Push the *qi* down from forehead to the chest to sinking the *qi* into the lower abdomen dantian.

Figure 1: Position of the Energy Points

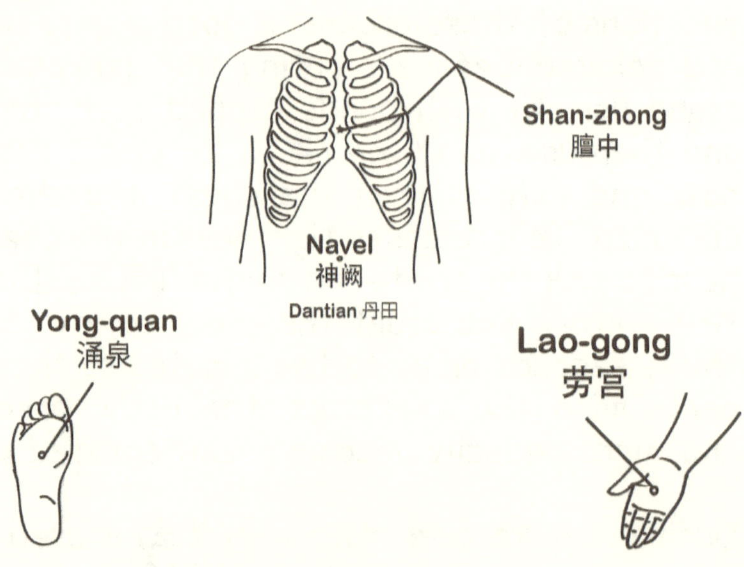

THE SEVEN EXERCISE REGIMENS

We always begin and end each exercise regimen standing upright with the feet together and the hands cupped (see figure 2, page 6 in Section I) for one to two minutes. This meditative posture keeps us physically relaxed and mentally calm for a while. Before starting, standing straight maintains a firm posture to ensure steadiness and strength so that we can go through the whole practice ensuring firm support from the spine. Upon closing the exercise, the moment of standing quietly allows the *qi* to move from the channels into the lower abdominal dantian to be stored.

Regimen 1 (Principal Regimen): Harmonising the Yin-Yang Energy *Qi*

This principal regimen imitates the take-off and landing action of the bean goose (大雁起落). The exercise involves hand and limb movements, raising and lowering of the body trunk, opening the palms facing upwards and pressing the palms down as we move downwards. '*Mind-will (意念)*' is also used to softly direct our concentration at the *lao-gong* (劳宫) acupressure point on the palm, the ten fingers and front of the body from above the head pushing the *qi* down the chest to sinking the *qi* into the lower abdomen dantian elixir field.

As the movements of this exercise are structured, rhythmic, and harmonious, it creates a relaxed feeling of general ease. The whole exercise harmonizes the yin-yang energy *qi*. When there is no excess or deficiency of one over the other, sickness does not prevail. From my master's clinical observations, he found that this regimen improves *qi* and blood circulation and that it has significant healing effects on abnormal blood pressure, lung infections, and poor digestion.

Figure Regimen 1 : (Principal Regimen) Harmonising the Yin-Yang Energy *Qi*

1. Ready
2. Breathe out
Slowly place bent knee above toes
Straighten both legs
3. Breathe in
To straighten the hind leg, stand on toes
4. Take a deep breath

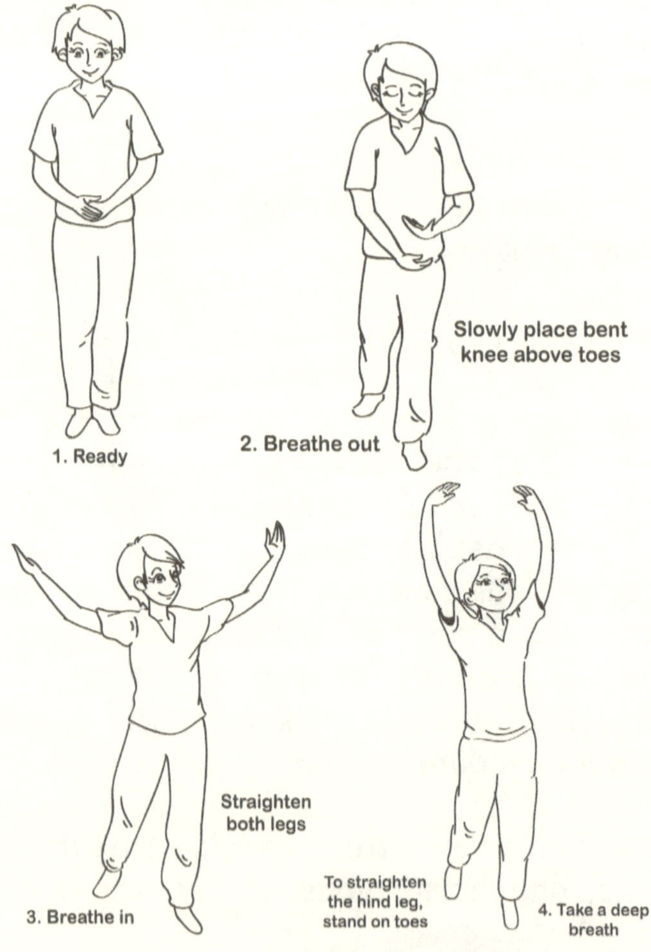

Turn palms
outwards
5. Slowly move
arms down
For balance, flex
the knee to put
weight on the heel
Ready to pull
in front leg
6. Breathe out
Slowly
Imagine sitting on a
chair. If the knee aches
do not sit too low
7. Breathe out
all the air

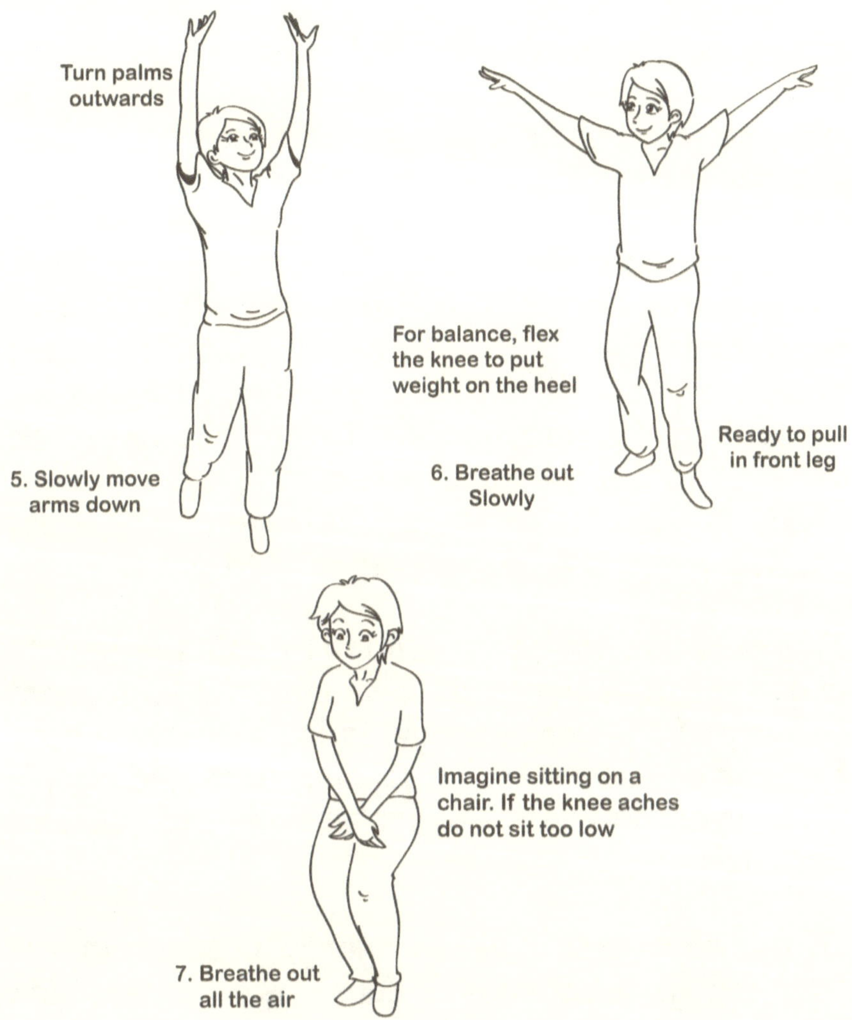

Regimen 2: Nurturing the Liver and Toning the Gallbladder

This regimen imitates the spreading out and folding of wings from front to back (前后展翅) of the bean goose to support and strengthen the function of the liver and gallbladder. The whole exercise is structured with smooth and flowing movements to create a relaxed feeling of general ease in movement of the head, neck, waist, legs, and hands. We begin by putting one leg forward, and letting the heel rest lightly on the ground with the toes tilted upward. This placing allows the primordial *qi* to enter the body through the *da-dun* (大敦) liver acupoint on the big toe. The hind leg with knee bent stays with foot firmly on the ground with the hip supporting the body weight. During the exercise, our eyes follow the hand movements, and '*mind-will (意念)*' is used to softly concentrate at the waist and the place where the liver is positioned.

This exercise has been found to be able to regulate *qi* and blood in the liver to subdue the exuberant activity of the yang energy. It is particularly good for women with menopause disorders and people with syndromes of hypertension and chronic hepatitis.

In addition, any adverse energy present in the liver and gallbladder may cause us to have sallow complexion, frequent desire to sigh or to take deep breaths, heavy head, dizziness, tired legs, a tendency to stumble, stiff muscles, and pain in the rib cage or waist, as well as tired eyes. The character *xu (嘘)* (pronounced in English as "she") is used to nurture the liver and tone the gallbladder to reduce these ailments.

Figure Regimen 2: Nurturing the Liver and Toning the Gallbladder

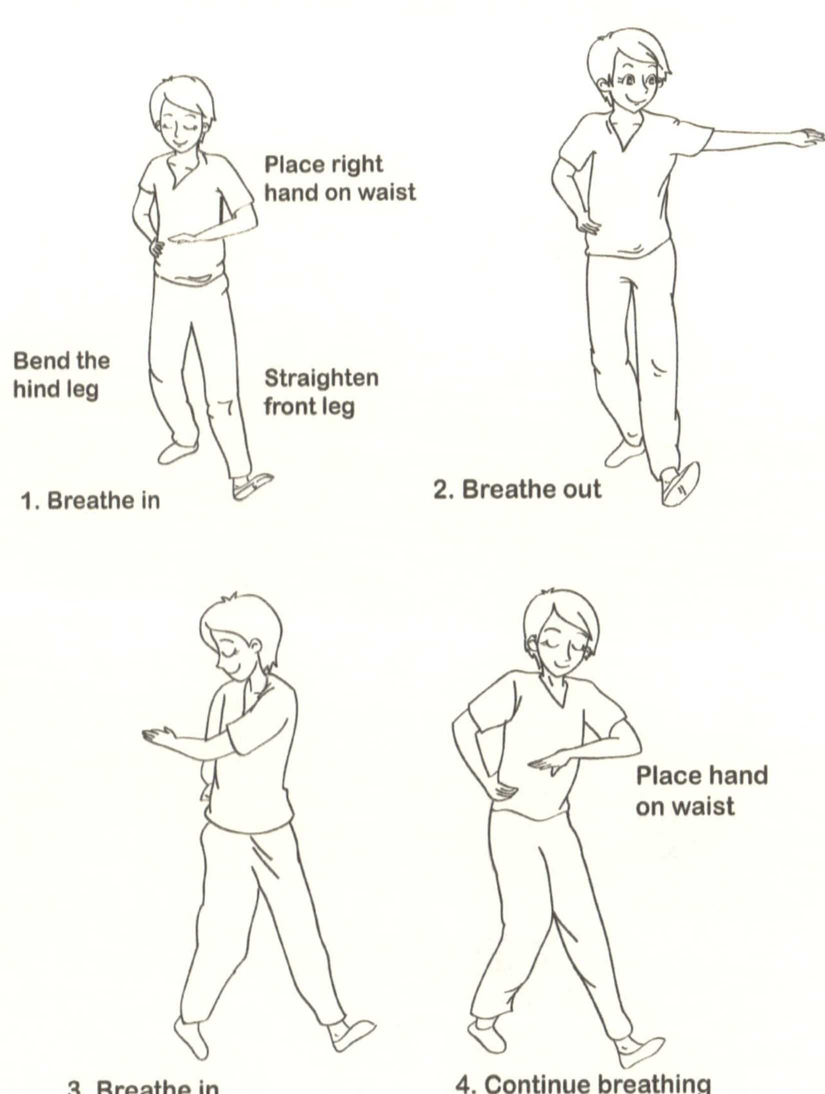

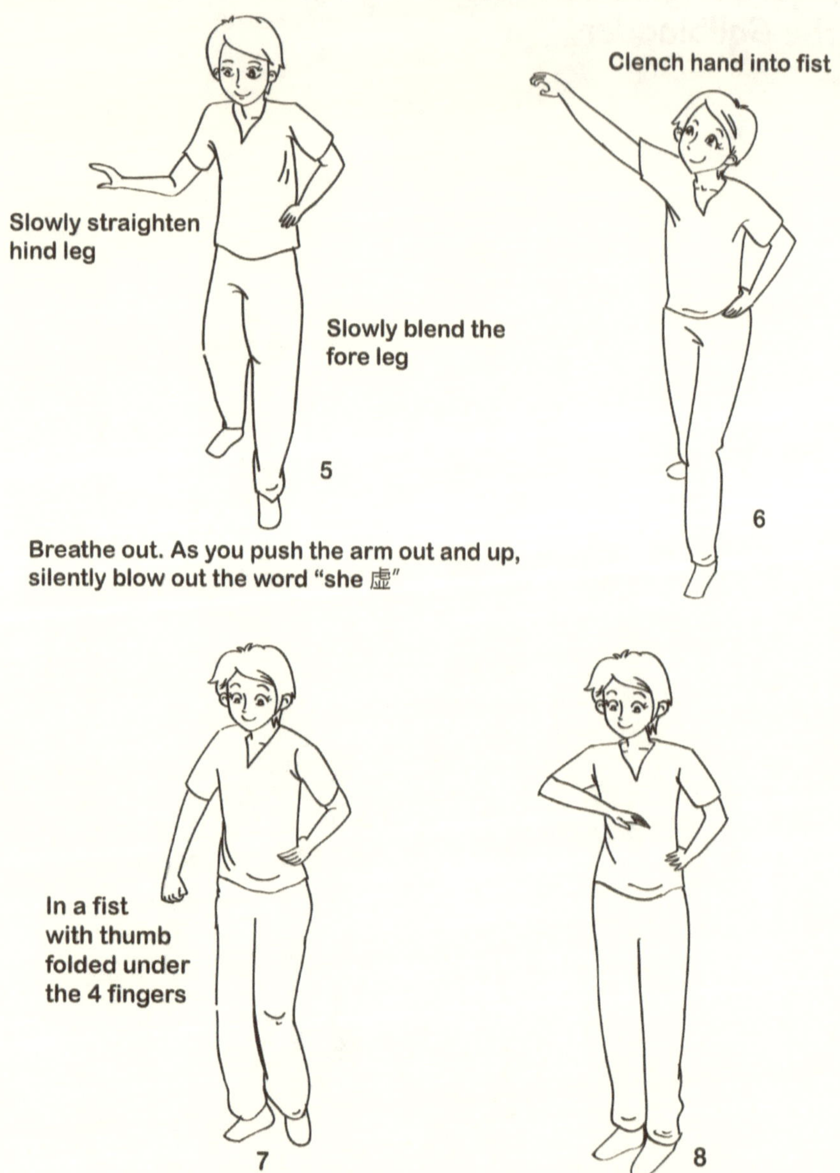

Breathe in as you pull down the arm and pull in the leg to stand feet together. Ready to start on the right

Regimen 3: Nourishing the Heart and Toning the Small Intestine

This regimen pays special attention to the movement of the head bending forth and back. In the knee-bending posture, we shift the body weight onto the buttocks. '*Mind-will (意念)*' is used softly to direct the breath to the *lao-gong* (劳宫) acupressure point on the palm, the *shan-zhong* (膻中) acupressure point on the chest, and then down the arm, palm to the tip of the little finger.

It has been found that this exercise can regulate *qi* and blood in the heart and small intestine, and it has significant therapeutic effect on coronary heart disease, rheumatic heart, palpitation, and insomnia.

In addition, any adverse energy present in these organs may cause us to have parched throat and violent thirst, sweaty palms, stiff forearm, pains in the neck, shoulder blade, dim eyesight, hardness of hearing, pains in the heart and back of the ears. We may feel cold but hot in the head, The character *ke (呵)* (pronounced in English as "ker") is used to nourish the heart and tone the small intestine to reduce these ailments.

Figure Regimen 3: Nourishing the Heart and Toning the Small Intestine

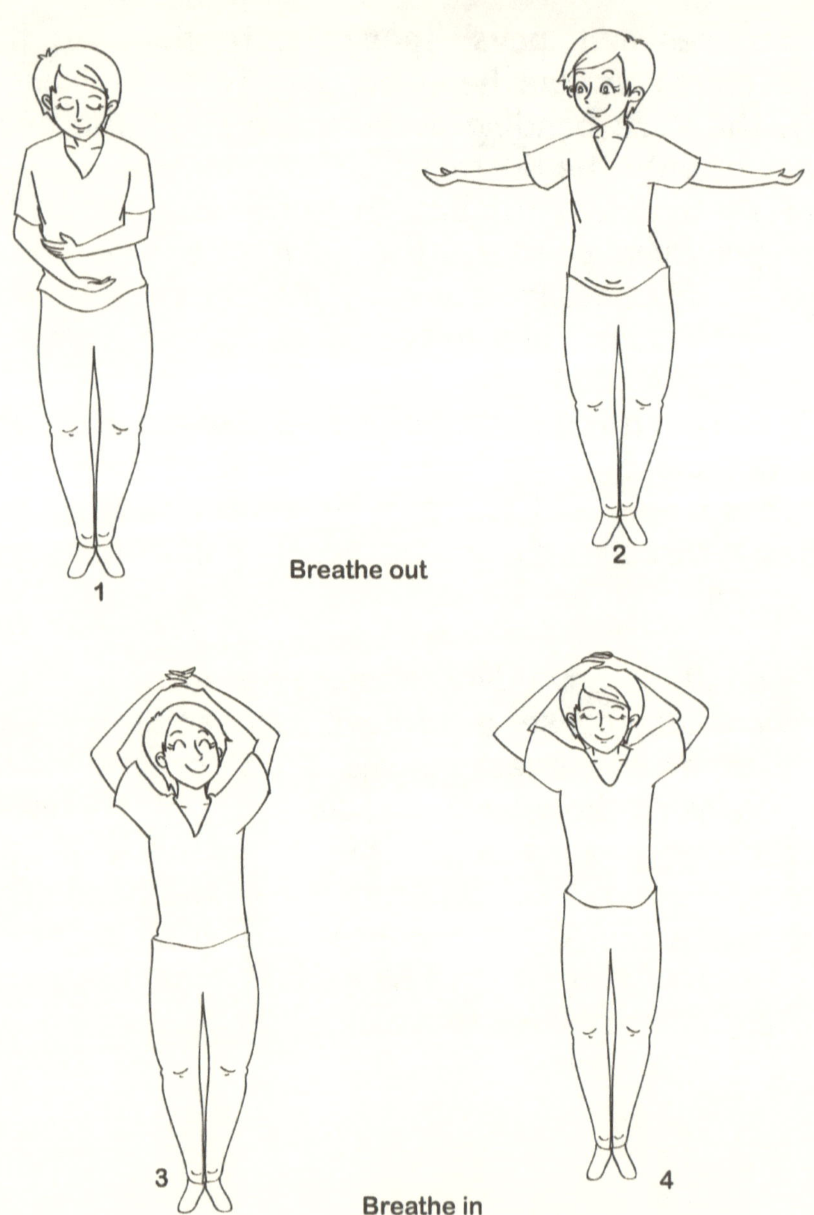

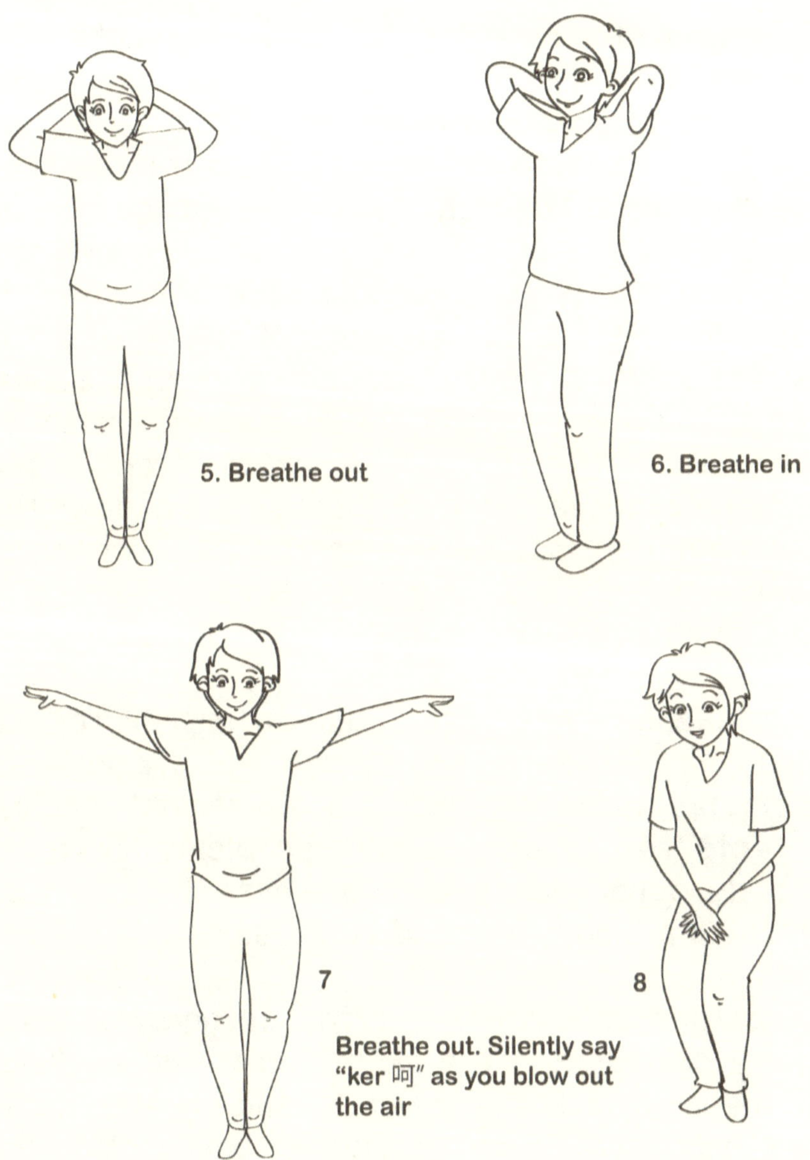
5. Breathe out
6. Breathe in
7
8
Breathe out. Silently say
"ker 呵" as you blow out
the air

Regimen 4: Invigorating the Spleen and Toning the Stomach

This regimen includes stretching the trunk, the legs, and the arms, flexing the elbow joints, exercising the wrist, folding the fingers into a fist and rotating the fist. The left foot moves left to the width of the shoulders. The right foot is placed squarely on the ground to support the body weight when the left foot is moved. When the body is lowered, it rests in a semi-squat position. '*Mind-will (意念)*' is used to softly direct our concentration at the navel or the abdomen, at *lao-gong* (劳宫) on the palm, at the knees or tips of the toes, and the front of the body from above the head, pushing the *qi* down the chest and sinking the *qi* into the lower abdomen dantian elixir field. The steadiness and grace in this regimen exudes calmness and tranquillity.

This exercise has been found to improve *qi* and blood circulation to the spleen and stomach. It promotes digestion and has significant healing effects for chronic gastric problems, gastritis and duodenal ulcers, and improves functions of the heart, lungs, liver and kidneys.

In addition, adverse energy in these organs may cause sticky dry taste in the mouth, pains and swellings of the knees, pains in the chest and breasts, heavy legs, and disability of the big toe. Saying aloud the character *hu (呼)* (pronounced in English as "hoo") gets rid of the adverse energy and invigorates the spleen and tone the stomach to reduce these ailments.

Figure Regimen 4:Invigorating the Spleen and Toning the Stomach

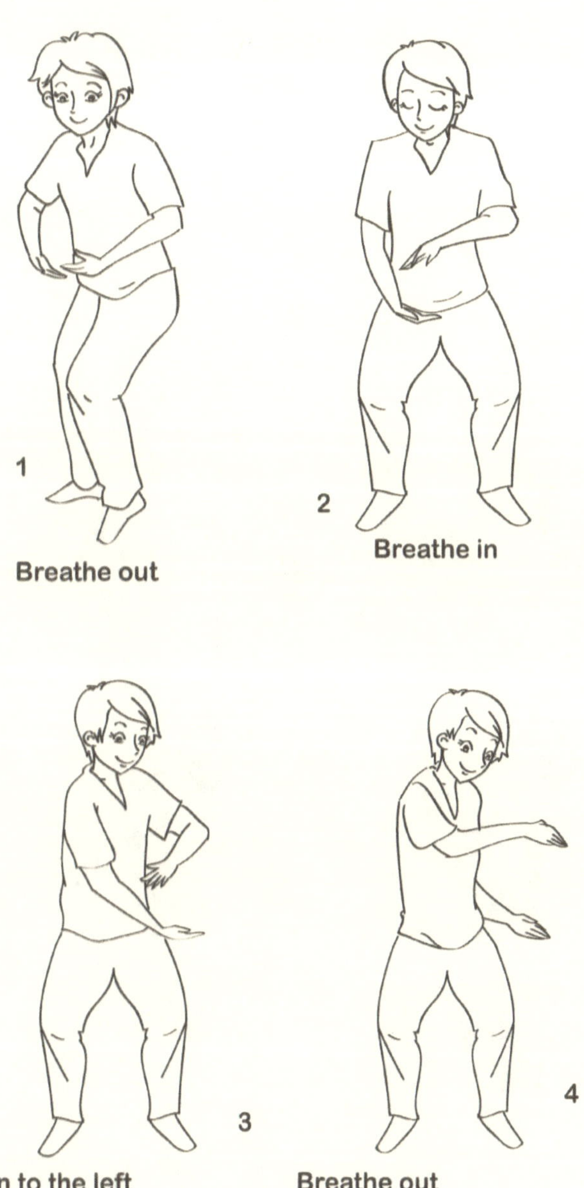

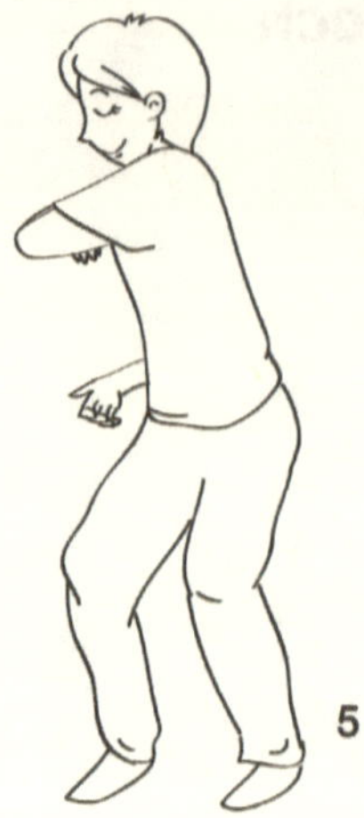

Place right arm on top and turn to the right.

Move up the left arm and turn body to the left with palm facing outward moving across the eyes.

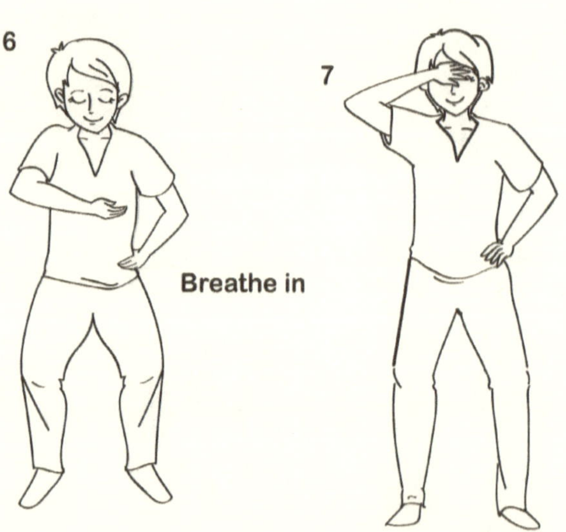

Breathe in

Continue to do

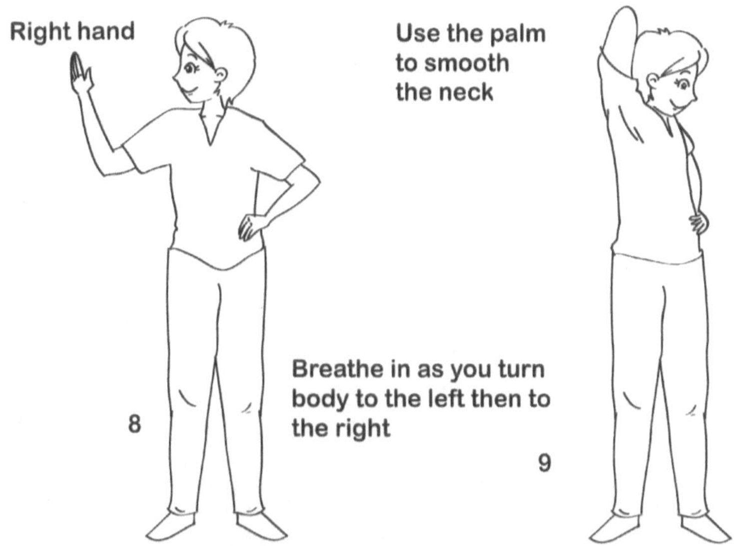

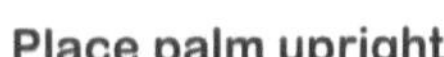

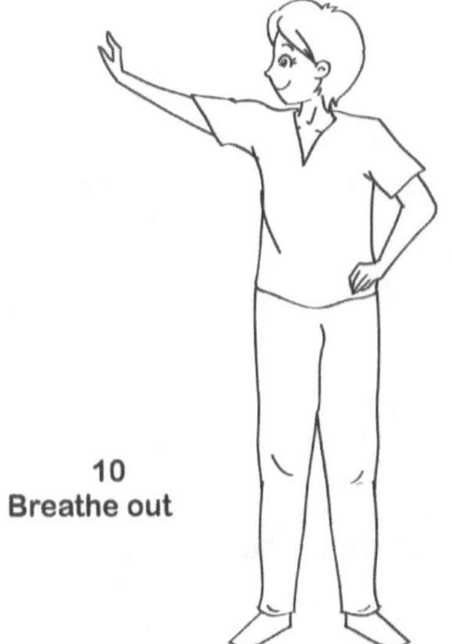

Palm to wrist at right angle

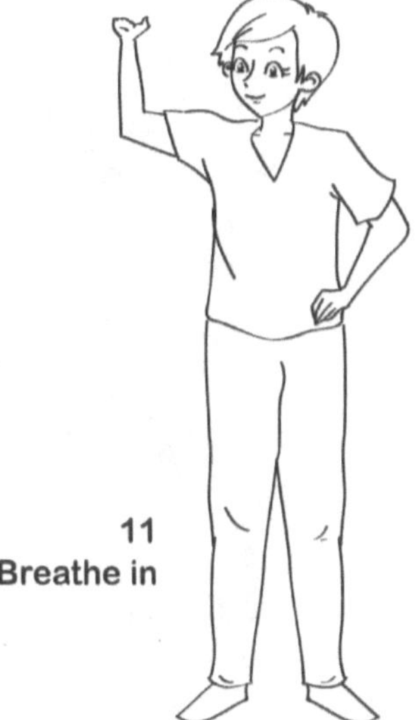

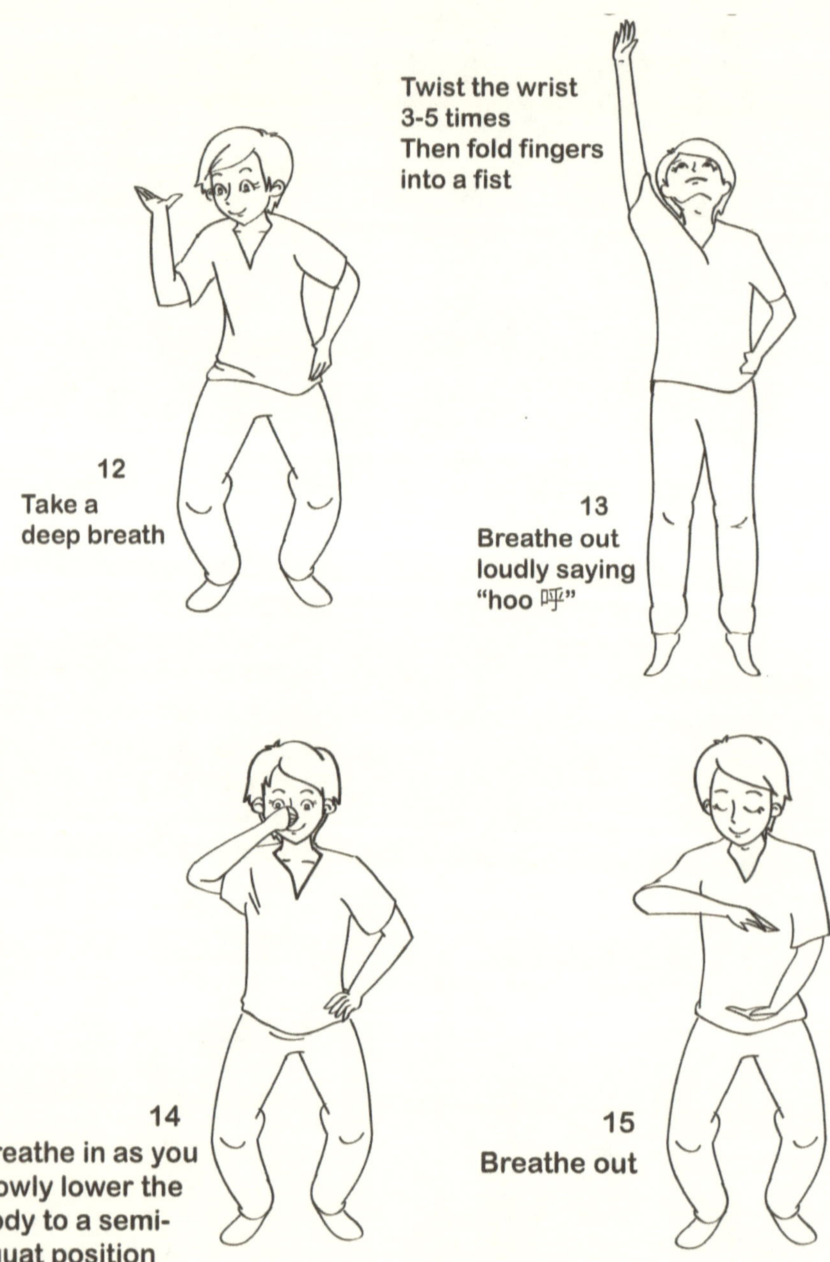
Twist the wrist
3-5 times
Then fold fingers
into a fist
12
Take a
deep breath
13
Breathe out
loudly saying
“hoo 呼”
14
Breathe in as you
slowly lower the
body to a semi-
squat position
15
Breathe out

Regimen 5: Moisturising the Lungs and Toning the Large Intestine

This regimen imitates the bean goose dipping its wings to splash water onto the body (大雁拍水) to support and strengthen functions of the lungs and large intestine. The whole exercise is structured with smooth and flowing movements to create a relaxed feeling of general ease in the movement of the head, legs, and arms. When moving one leg forward, bend the knee above the toes. The hind leg stays at the same spot, with the foot firmly on the ground and with the hip supporting the body weight. During the exercise, our eyes follow the hand movements and '*mind-will (意念)*' is used to softly concentrate at the arm, at *shan-zhong* (膻中) on the chest and stomach, and at tip of the thumb and index finger.

This exercise has been found to improve *qi* and blood circulation into the lungs and large intestine. It promotes greater intake of oxygen and has significant healing effects for coughs and colds, asthma, and fatigue from overwork.

In addition, adverse energy in these organs may give us tight muscles, a tight chest, no strength in the thumb, index finger, and below the hips, headaches, shoulder pain, itchy skin, congested nasal passage, phlegm from the bronchi, coughing, susceptibility to colds, and constipation. Saying the character *si (四)* gets rid of the adverse energy to moisturise the lungs and tone the large intestine to reduce these ailments.

Figure Regimen 5: Moisturising the Lungs and Toning the Large Intestine

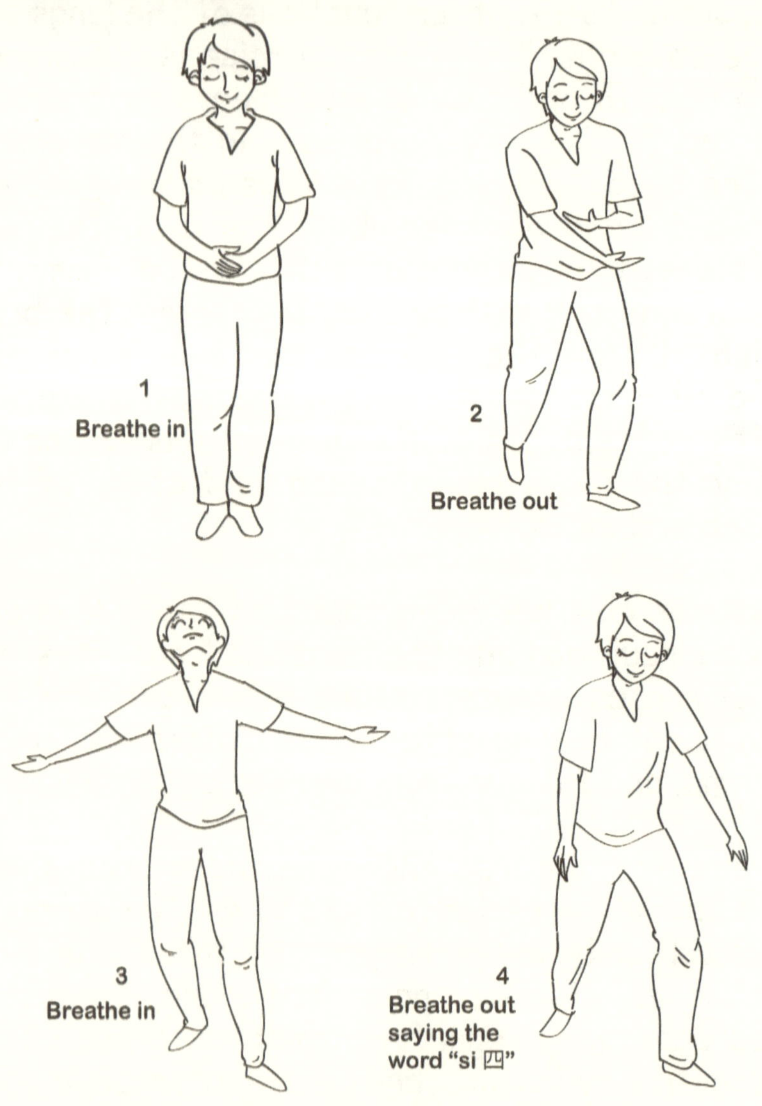

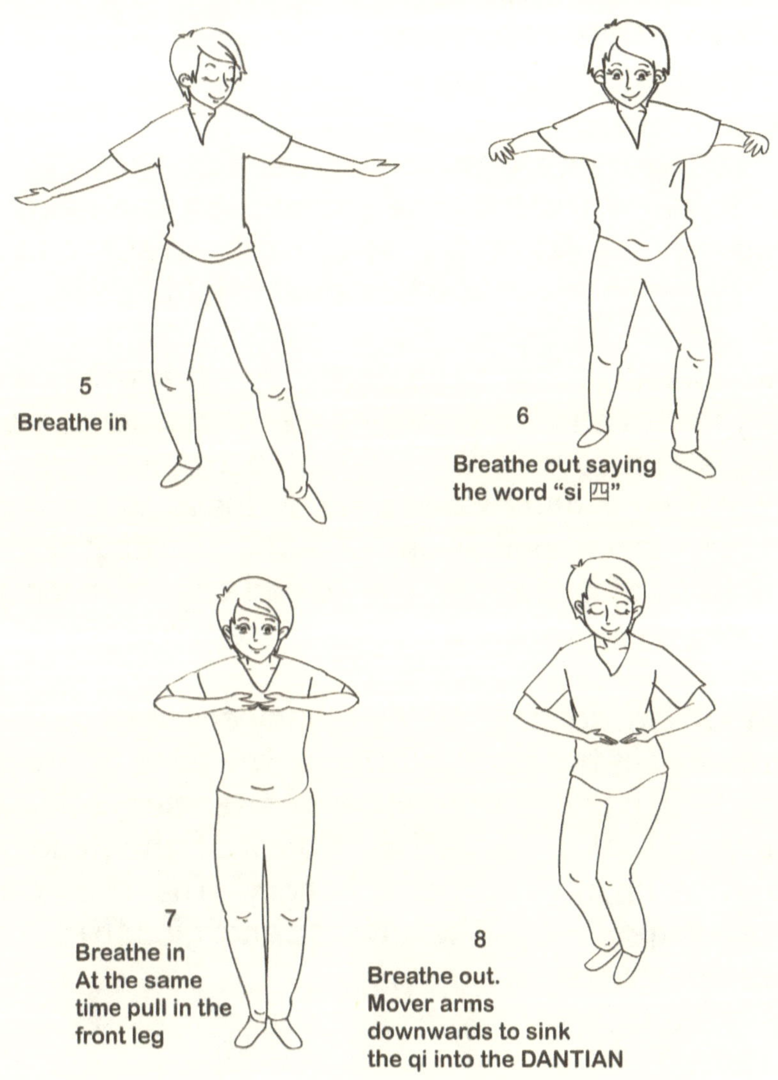
5
Breathe in
6
Breathe out saying
the word "si 四"
7
Breathe in
At the same
time pull in the
front leg
8
Breathe out.
Mover arms
downwards to sink
the qi into the DANTIAN

Regimen 6: Strengthening the Kidneys and Toning the Urinary Bladder

This regimen involves turning the trunk to the back and then returning to the front. Then bend forward and then backward. During the exercise, our eyes follow the movements and '*mind-will (意念)*' is used softly to concentrate at the area of the spine nearest to the kidneys, at the heel, at *yong-quan* (涌泉) at the soles of the feet, and at the lower abdomen dantian elixir field.

This exercise has been found to strengthen the yang energy and increase *jing* (精), the essence fluid that is our foundation for life in the kidneys. By circulating *qi* and blood to the kidneys and urinary bladder, it has significant effect on strengthening functions of the brain, the sexual organs, improve hearing and normalise irregular menstruation.

In addition, adverse energies may cause us to have heaviness in the head, ringing in the ears, frequent urination, pains in the hollow of the knee, calf and foot, backache, headache at back of the head, no appetite in spite of being hungry, The character *chui (吹)* gets rid of the adverse energies to reduce these ailments.

Figure Regimen 6: Strengthening the Kidneys and Toning the Urinary Bladder

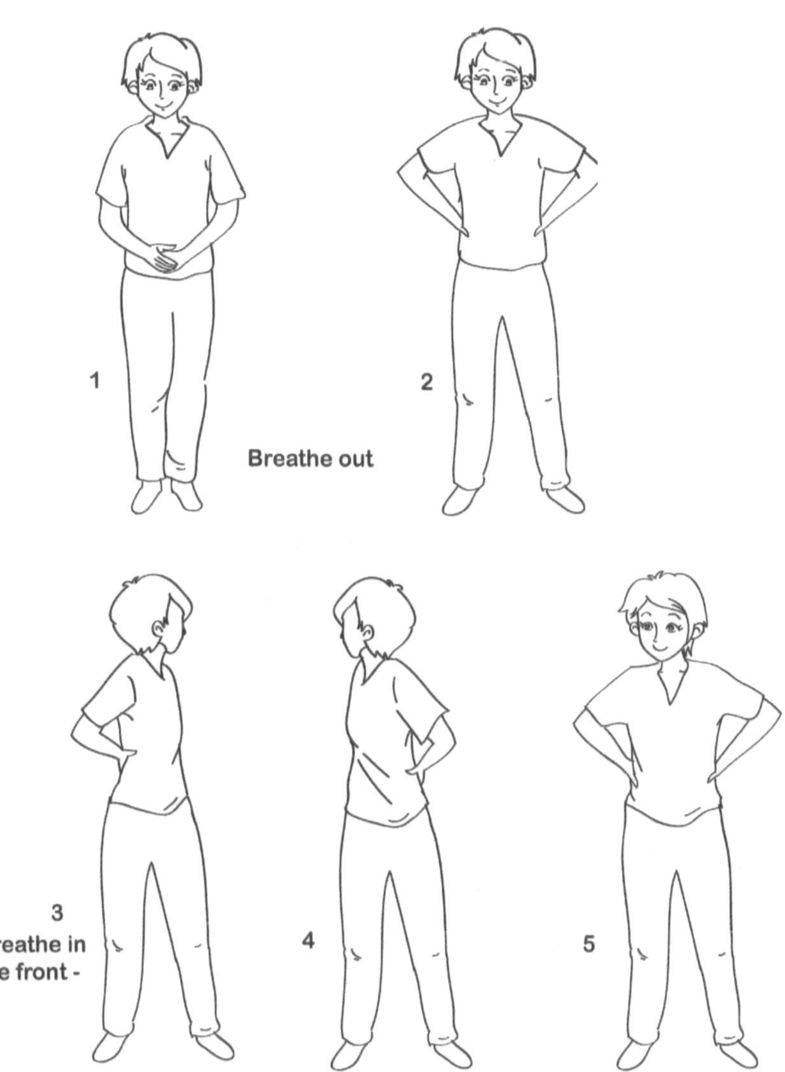

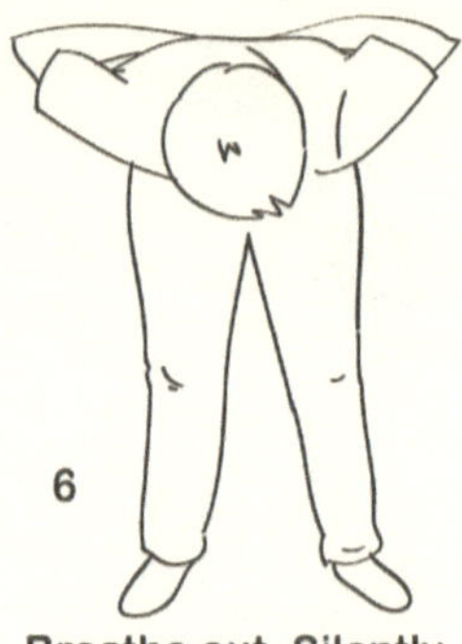

6

Breathe out. Silently
say the word "chui 吹"

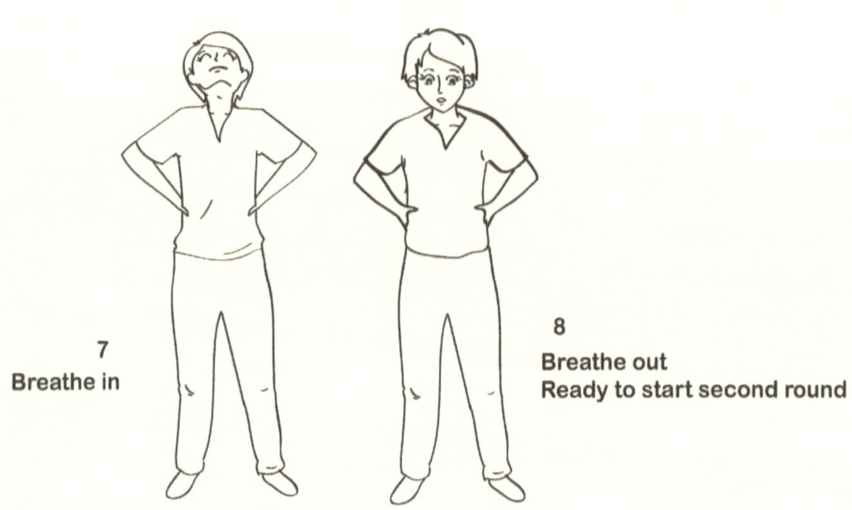

7
Breathe in

8
Breathe out
Ready to start second round

Regimen 7: Regulating the Triple-Heater Sequentially and Supporting the Functions of the Lymphatic and Endocrine Systems

This regimen imitates the bean goose looking left and right before taking flight (左右看足). It has in it the all-inclusive set of six positions—turning left and right, looking forward then backward, and moving upward then downward. The whole exercise is structured. It involves moving one leg forward and bending the knee above the toes. The hind leg stays at the same spot with the foot firmly on the ground and with the hip supporting the body weight. There are also movements to exercise the eyes, head, neck, the four limbs, ankles, waist, abdomen and the spine.

'*Mind-will (意念)*' is used to concentrate softly at the *lao-gong* (劳宫) in the centre of the palm, the tip of the ring finger, the back of the heel, and the forehead. Then from the forehead, push the *qi* down the chest passing the upper and middle dantian all the way down, sinking the *qi* into the lower dantian elixir field. The steadiness and grace of this regimen exudes calmness and tranquillity.

Although the flowing, smooth, graceful, elegant movements of this regimen outwardly look fluid, it has been found that in reality it possesses an internal strength to regulate the triple-heater (upper, middle, and lower *dantian* (丹田)) and is able to support and strengthen the functions of the lymphatic and endocrine systems. The change in positions improves *qi* and blood circulation to the entire body, all the way to the tips of the fingers and toes. This regimen has significant healing effects for people with water retention in their body systems, and abnormal functions of their kidneys, lungs, liver, spleen and stomach.

In addition, adverse energies may cause frequent low blood pressure, poor circulation, heavy head, loose gums, sensitive to temperature change, allergy or rashes. The character formula *xi (嘻)* (pronounced in English as "see") is used to get rid of the adverse energies.

Figure Regimen 7: Regulating the Triple-Heater (理三焦) Sequentially and Supporting the Functions of the Lymphatic and Endocrine Systems

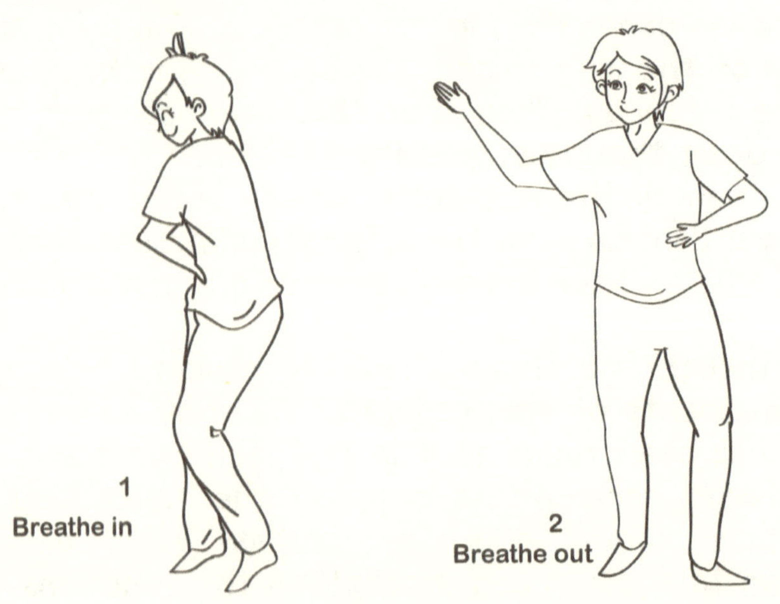

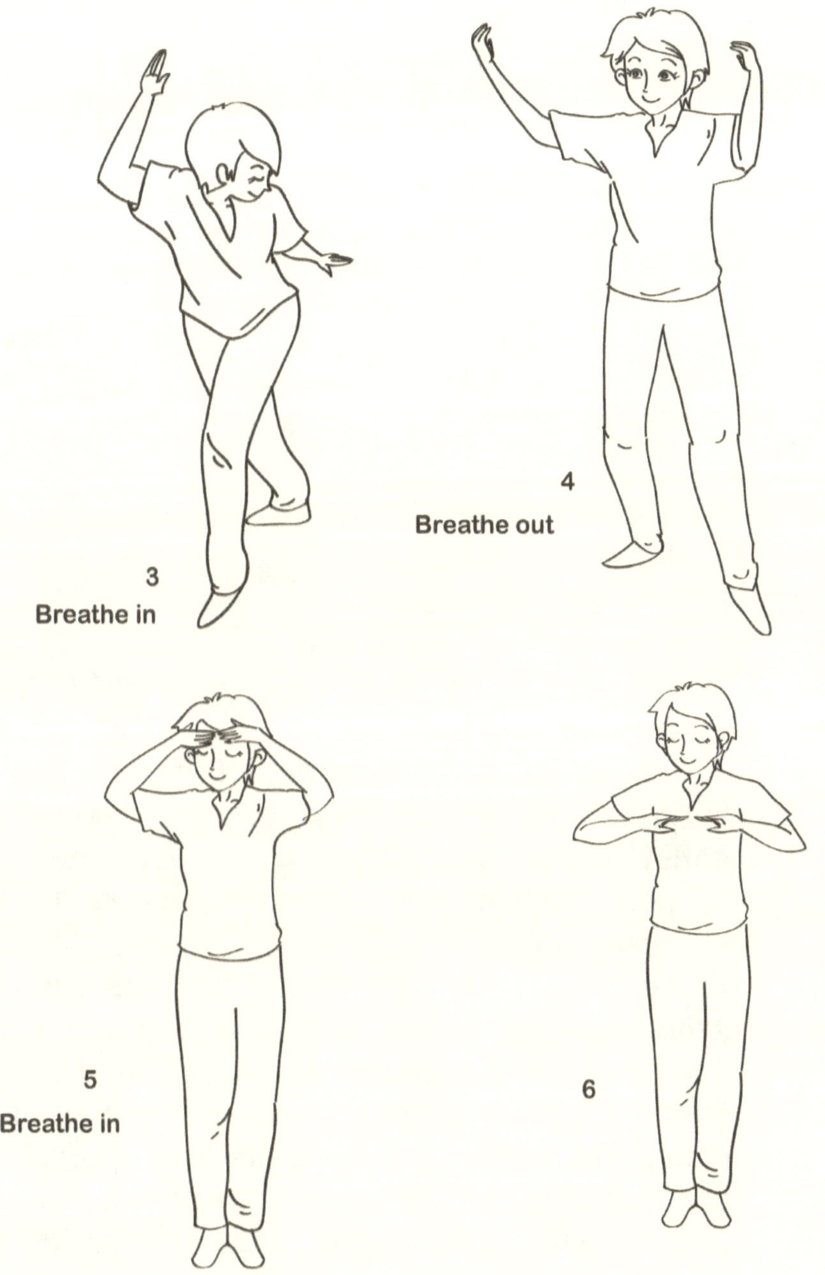
3
Breathe in
4
Breathe out
5
Breathe in
6

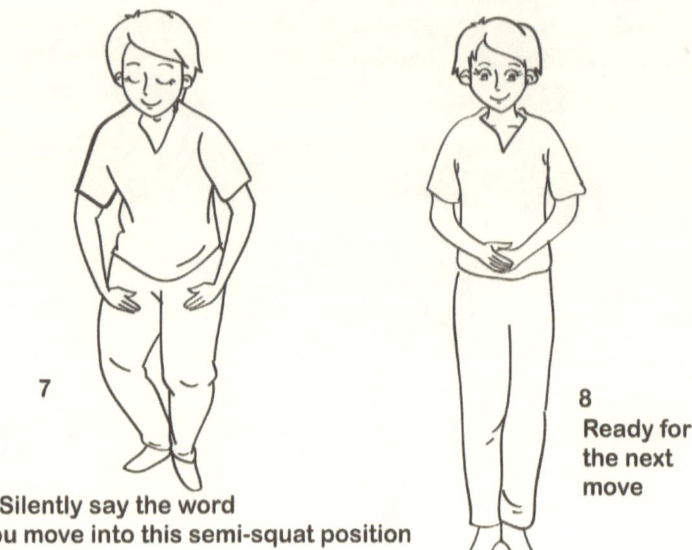

POINTS TO NOTE

1. When practising *da yan liu zi gong* (大雁六字功), one normal session for the seven regimens would take about thirty to forty minutes. We must know our own physical constitution—old or young, in good health or poor health—and adapt the exercise to our own needs. For those of us who decide to do one or two regimens a day, instead of stopping after seven rounds, we can increase our exercise for each regimen up to twelve rounds, left and right being counted as one round. In general, the number of exercise regimens we choose to do each day must give us comfort and relaxation, not exhaustion.

2. Before starting, make sure there are no physical and mental tensions. The body and mind should be fully relaxed to allow a smooth flow of the energy *qi*. Remember to do the standing meditation for at least thirty seconds or up to two minutes.

3. The speed of the movements and the level of raising the limbs must be without physical exertion. Doing the exercises hastily can be harmful.

4. As a beginner, you may sometimes feel some discomfort, but you should not give up or rapidly change to another form of Qigong from another school. Rapid change to other forms can be unsettling to the *qi* and may produce uncomfortable side effects.

   (From my own experience, I can say that to be able to enjoy the benefits of *da-yan-liu-zi-gong* (大雁六字功), you need to practise regularly once a day for at least six months to realize its therapeutic effects.)

5. In meditation, we draw on mind-will (意念) to cause internal *qi* to move out of the *dantian (丹田)* and circulate in the energy *qi* channels. There is internal activity while in a state of stillness. In *da yan liu zi gong (大雁六字功)*, we resort to '*mind-will (意念)*' and breathing

disciplines and to external movements of the limbs and body to conduct the internal *qi* to flow. There is internal tranquillity while being externally active.

Veteran Qigong masters often stressed that if we wanted a holistic effect in our practices, we should do both tranquil and mobile Qigong. From the exercises given in this book, it would mean that we ought to do meditation and *da yan liu zi gong (大雁六字功)*, at each single practice.

6. Drink a glass of warm water before starting on the exercise.

7. Do not concentrate too hard on the breathing. Breathe naturally (normal exhalation and inhalation) with eyes following the hand movements. When the breathing is natural and smooth and the upper part of the body (head and chest) is free of tightness and congestion, the *qi* will sink down to the dantian elixir field in the lower abdomen.

Dos and Don'ts During the Practice of Da Yan Liu Zi Gong (大雁六字功)

To avoid any side effects, pay particular attention to the Dos and Don'ts

The Dos

- Adhere strictly to the prescribed exercise regimens.
- Keep the body relaxed. Half an hour before the exercise, stop all strenuous activities to prepare for a calm and restful mind.
- Achieve a state of "letting go" of all thoughts before starting on the practice. (Do a standing meditation one to two minutes according to your needs.)
- Look cheerful by wearing a smile throughout the practice. Put aside fretful or anxious thoughts. If such thoughts are disturbing, stop the practice, go for a walk or take a rest or do other things until you feel more at ease.

The Don'ts

- Don't rush through the exercise.
- Don't think of other things.

- Don't have an empty or full stomach. Avoid eating very cold or hot food, or spicy food before the exercise.
- Don't end your exercise abruptly.
- Don't stand facing the sun or the wind.

NORMAL AND ABNORMAL EFFECTS EXPERIENCED IN *DA YAN LIU ZI GONG* (大雁六字功)

The normal and abnormal effects listed below may or may not be felt by everyone at the same time in the same manner. We are all individuals. We live through life differently. We may not be experiencing the same physical, mental, and spiritual problems at the time of practice. Remember not to chase after effects. Let things take their natural course.

Normal Effects

1. Feeling a sense of general ease and restfulness.
2. Sweating a little.
3. Feeling less mental and physical fatigue. Sleeping more soundly.
4. Improved appetite.

5. Sensing a tingling sensation under the skin and at the extremities of the fingers—a sign of *qi* circulating the *qi* channels.

6. Feeling vigorously healthy.

Abnormal Effects

1. Increased heart beat and breathlessness.
   Remedy: Relax your movements, breathe softly and slowly, and ensure your posture is correct.

2. Dry mouth and itchy throat.
   Remedy: Do not breathe with the mouth open too widely or closed too tightly; drink a little warm water before practising.

3. There is a feeling of abdominal distension. This means the qi is travelling the opposite way—from the abdomen up to the chest.
   Remedy: Soften the concentration, breathe slowly and softly, and ensure your posture is correct.

4. There is a feeling of mental confusion with haziness.
   Remedy: Soften the concentration, breathe slowly and softly, and move slowly.

5. Headache.
   Remedy: Relax the muscles, breathe slowly and softly, and ensure your posture is correct.

EXERCISES TO RELIEVE DISCOMFORT

In normal circumstances, if we pay attention and follow the requisites and adhere to doing the prescribed movements in each exercise regimen correctly, no serious deviations will surface. Most are discomforts caused by anxiety and tension and can be relieved by doing one or two of the following *qi* regulation and relaxation exercises.

The *Qi* Regulation Method (调气法)

Most discomforts upset the smooth flow of the internal *qi* in the body. By doing this exercise, the internal *qi* is activated to move in a regular cycle to correct any imbalance in the *qi* function. This exercise relieves such discomforts as fatigue, inability to sleep, feeling tired and weak after an illness, or going through mental confusion with a hazy feeling.

To help achieve the best results when practising, remember to maintain a relaxed upright posture, a regulatory form of light, smooth breathing and a calm and restful mind free of distracting thoughts.

The Exercise

Before starting or closing this exercise, always have your hands **placed either by the side or** cupped over the navel to nurture the dantian elixir field. Stand with the feet together or apart in a meditative manner. Breathe lightly and naturally for two minutes to allow the mind to become calm and restful. After the closing and before you walk away, blow out all the air from the lungs by saying aloud *hu (呼)* (pronounced in English as "hoo").

Do the exercise as shown in figure 2. Repeat the exercise seven to nine times.

Figure 2: The *Qi* Regulation Exercise

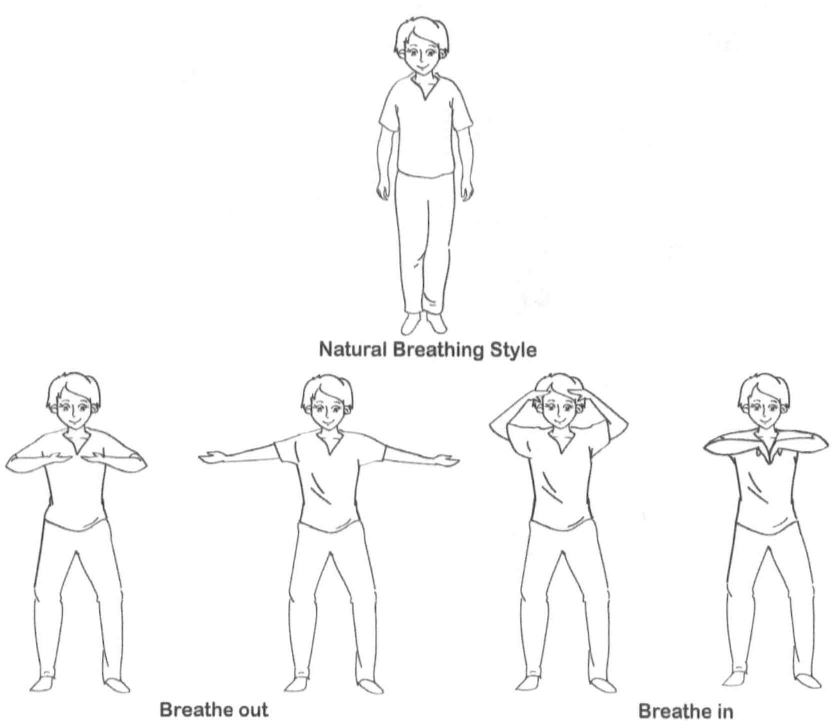

The Tapping Exercise

This exercise tones the body muscles and removes clots along the *qi* channels and collaterals to stimulate the smooth flow of *qi*. When you are feeling downhearted or have a tense feeling in your muscles, tapping lightly along the designed path of the body with the palms or fingers of the hands will help in relieving the discomforts.

Tapping Procedure

To help achieve best results when practising, remember to maintain a relaxed, upright posture, natural breathing and use '*mind-will (意念)*' to follow the path of tapping.

To begin, rub the hands until they are warm. Then lightly tap. Repeat each segment of tapping three times to a count of seven.

Figure 3: Tapping Exercise

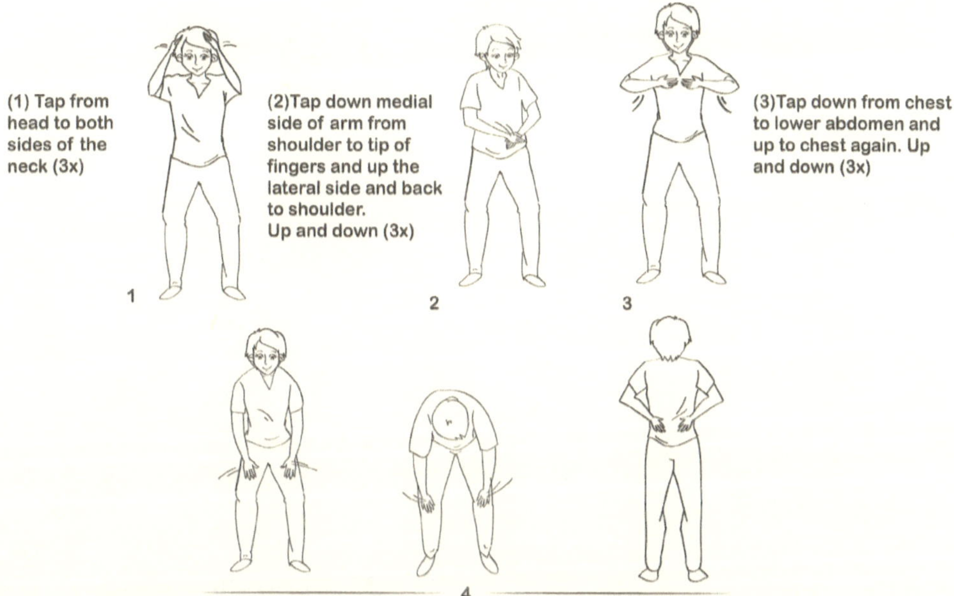

Free-Walking

Should you feel any uneasiness or apprehension during the practices, stop for a few days to do twenty minutes or more of the walking exercises. There are two forms of walking we can choose to do: relaxed walking and '***mind-will (意念)***' walking.

In relaxed walking, simply look at the green scenery around you or listen to birds' and insects' calls as you walk

Figure 4: '*Mind-will (意念)*' Walking

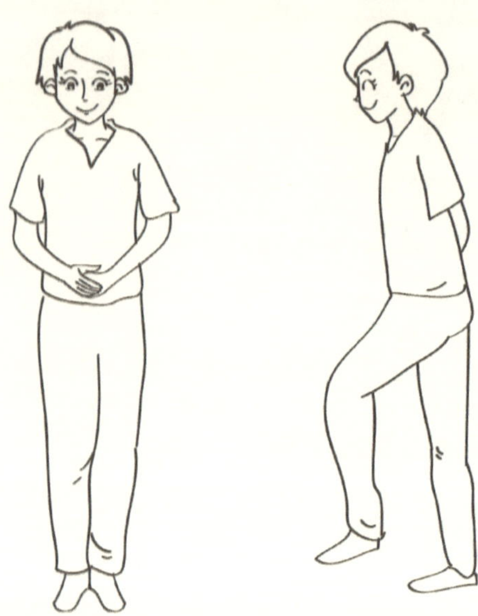

Before you start '*mind-will (意念)*' walking, calm the mind by standing still for thirty seconds to two minutes with the hands cupped over the navel. Begin by keeping your mind on the foot—one foot at a time. Start with the left foot, then the right.

Slowly lift your leg off the ground while inhaling through the nose, and move it slowly forward. Then slowly place the foot in front on the ground—toes first, then heel—while exhaling through the mouth.

Direct '*mind-will (意念)*' to the leg-foot movement; do not think of the breathing. Walk for ten minutes, and then continue with relaxed walking for as long as you wish.

Section Three

Self-Massage With Acupressure

A Self-Aid Tool That Is Easy To Manage

UNDERSTANDING SELF-MASSAGE WITH ACUPRESSURE

Self-massage with acupressure exercises has elements of Qigong therapeutic approaches to stimulating the energy *qi* and blood to move to specific parts of the body that are troubling us. By applying soft massage and pressure on the acupoints (acupuncture-points), we develop a comfortable, warm, tingling sensation and a feeling of relaxation. These are signals telling us *qi* is moving.

Different exercises have different therapeutic functions and effects. The detailed layout makes it easy for us to select the appropriate form to suit our health conditions. The positive effects of massage and acupressure on healthcare are built up gradually. We do not need to wait till illness occurs. If we practise all the exercises regularly, we can help ourselves maintain a healthy constitution through the years.

Our massage tools are the palms, thumbs, fingers, and knuckles. Use them the correct way. They are effective for quick relief to specific ailments.

Massage with acupressure exercises can be practised as a cluster or individually. When selecting an individual exercise, it is better to do the head and face exercises in the early morning after waking up. As for the kidney exercise, do it before going to sleep. It helps with sleeping soundly through the night.

Our Massage Tools

Our massage tools are the fleshy part of our fingers and thumbs, the palms and knuckles. Take note of the right and wrong way to use them.

Figure 1: Our Massage Tools

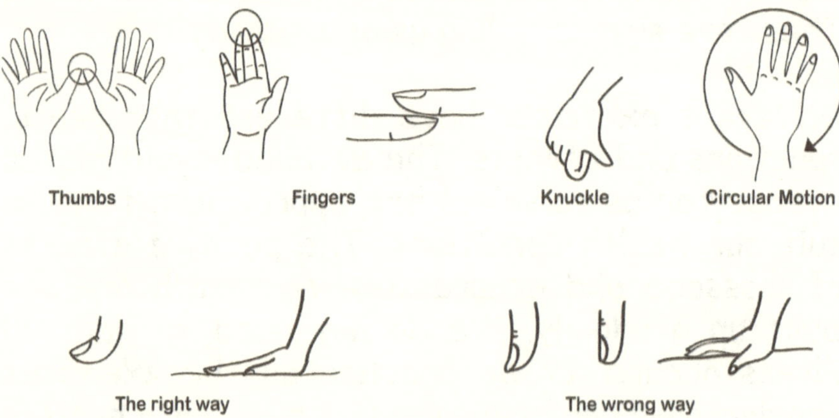

PROCEDURES

Head Exercise (头功)

Application Figure 1

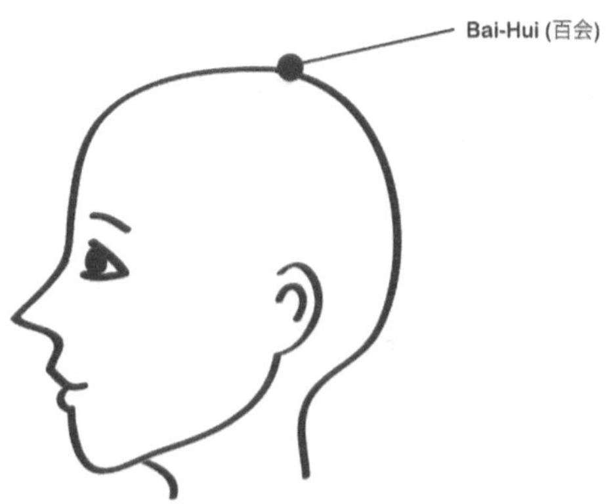

Massage and Acupressure Procedures:

1. Place the two **middle fingers** (one on top the other) lightly on acupoint *bai-hui* (百会). Press and knead the acupoint nine to eighteen times. Then pat lightly with one palm.

2. Interlock the fingers, and then push the palms across forehead 9-18 times

3. Comb through the hair with the fingers (not the nails) 9-18 times from front to back

Therapeutic Functions:

- *Activates flow of energy qi and blood to the head.*
- Promotes clear thinking.
- Prevents/treats headache and dizziness.

Nape of Neck Exercise (项功)

Application Figure 2

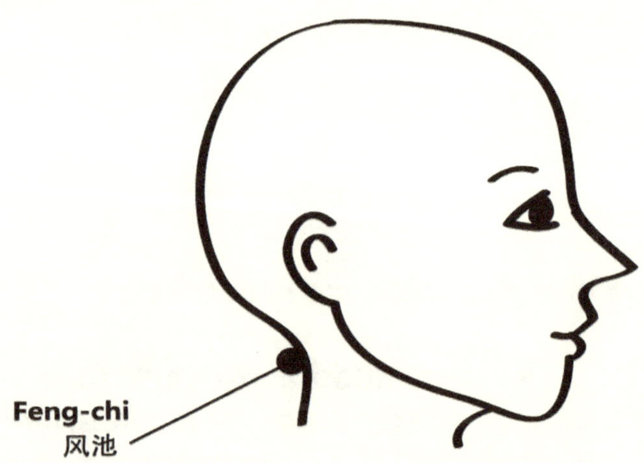

Massage and Acupressure Procedures:

1. Push the left and right palms alternately across the nape of the neck 9-18 times
2. Place the thumbs lightly on acupoint *feng-chi* (风池). Press and knead the acupoint 9-18 times.
3. Clasp the nape of the neck with interlocked fingers and tilt the head lightly backward with eyes looking upward. Repeat actions 3-5 times.

Therapeutic Functions:

- Activates flow of energy *qi* and blood to the neck.
- Relaxes neck muscles and tendons.
- Activates clear thinking.
- Prevents/treats headache, influenza, and stiff neck.

Face Exercise (面功-浴面)

Application Figure 3

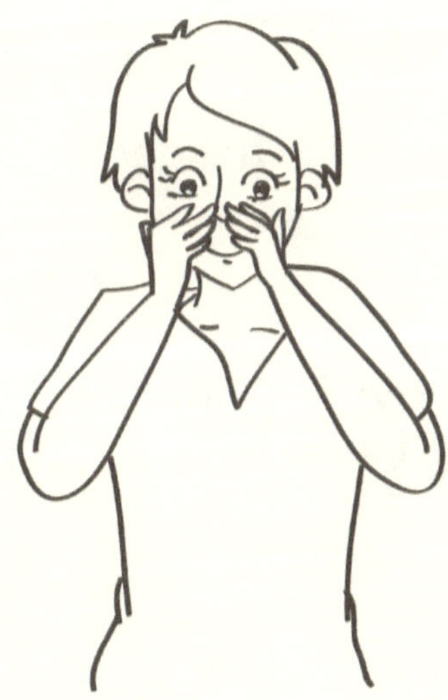

Massage Procedure:

1. Rub both hands together till warm. Lightly push the middle fingers up and down the sides of the nose 9-18 times

2. Use the middle fingers to push lightly up the sides of the nose until both palms are placed on the forehead. Move the palms sideways down the face to the chin. Then push the middle fingers up the sides of the lips and nose to the forehead again. Repeat the movement 9-18 times.

Therapeutic Functions:

- Activates the flow of energy *qi* and blood to the face.
- Promotes a ruddy and lustrous complexion.
- Eliminates wrinkles.
- Prevents/treats headache, dizziness, and stuffy nose.

Teeth and Tongue Exercise (齿功-叩击) (舌功)

Application Figure 4

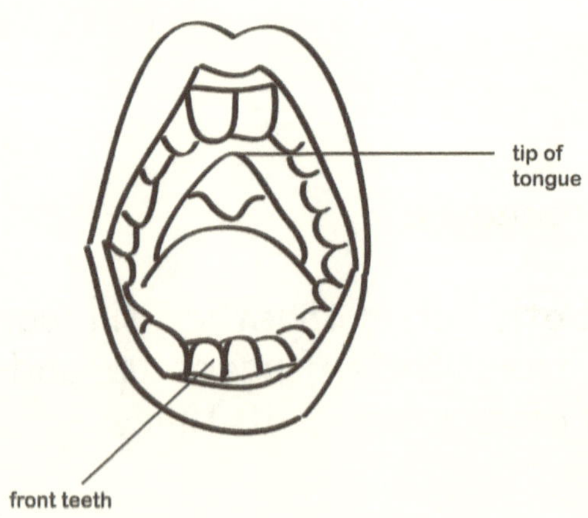

Massage Procedures:

Teeth:

1. Tap the upper molars onto the lower molars 9-18 times.

2. Tap the upper front teeth onto lower front teeth 9-18 times

3. Grind the molars 9-18 times.

4. Grip the teeth with the mouth closed for as long as you wish. (Breathe naturally. Focus the mind on the teeth.)

Tongue:

1. Roll the tip of the tongue to massage the front and then at the back of the teeth from top to bottom in a circular motion 6 times.

2. Place the tip of the tongue at the back part of the palate. Roll the tongue in a circular motion from top to bottom 9-18 times.

3. Swallow the saliva in three gulps, visualising it moving down the front body into the lower abdomen *dantian* (丹田) elixir field.

Therapeutic Functions:

- Calms the mind.
- Activates the flow of saliva.
- Strengthens the roots of the teeth.
- Aids digestion.
- The knocking and grinding of the teeth consolidate primordial *qi*.
  Do the grinding and gripping of the teeth during urination and defecation to help in streaming off all the urine from the bladder and smoothly move the bowels without any straining.

Nose Exercise (鼻功)

Application Figure 5

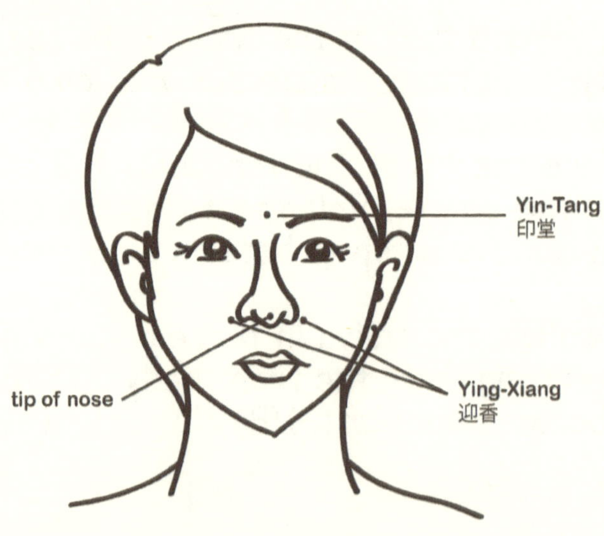

Massage and Acupressure Procedures:

1. Rub the side of the nose up and down in a flowing motion with the knuckles or fingers 9-18 times.

2. Press the middle and ring fingers against both sides of the nose with a light pressure 6 times.

3. Place the palm of one hand in a straight line from the *yin-tang* acupoint down to the tip of the nose. Then press, knead, and pressure 9-18 times the *yin-tang* (印堂) acupoint and the tip of the nose.

4. Press, knead, and pressure the *ying-xiang* (迎香) acupoint 9-18 times with the knuckle of the thumb or index finger.

Therapeutic Functions:

- Activates the flow of *qi* and blood to the mucus membrane of the nose and the lungs
- Prevents/treats the common cold, running nose, and nasal congestion.
- Relieves insomnia.

Eye Exercise (眼功)

Application Figure 6

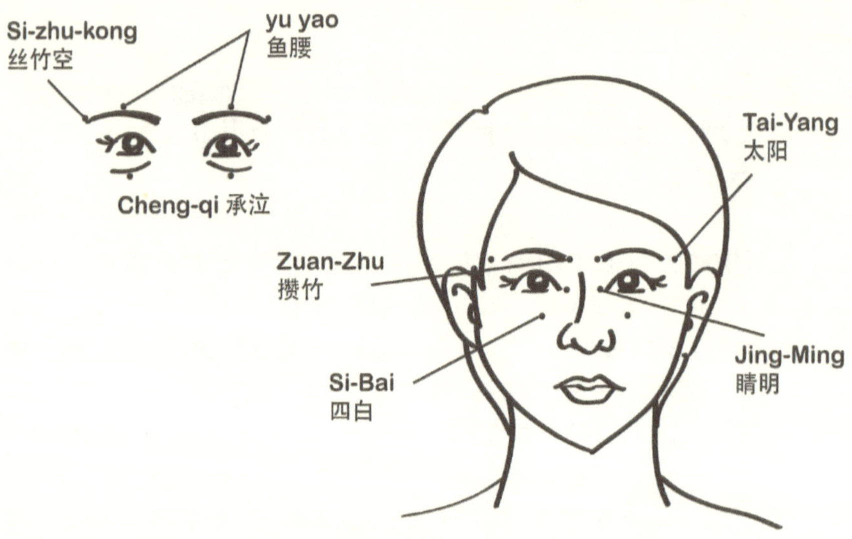

Massage and Acupressure Procedures:

1. Push with one knuckle 9-18 times along the upper and lower edges of the sockets of the eye in the direction of a reclining 8 (∞).

2. Lightly press, knead, pressure or push each of the following acupoints:

    - *jing-ming* (睛明)
    - *zuan-zhu* (攒竹)
    - *yu-yao* (鱼腰)
    - *si-zhu-kong* (丝竹空)

- *si-bai* (四白)
- *cheng-qi* (承泣)
- *tai-yang* (太阳)

3. Look fixedly at the tip of the nose to a count of 9 and then at a distant spot about five metres away, also to a count of 9. Do this alternately 6 times or more.

4. Rub the palms together until warm. Cover the eyes (slightly closed) with the palms. Lightly rub the eyes in the direction of a reclining 8 (∞) clockwise and then counter-clockwise 9-18 times.

5. Nurture the eyes. Close the eyes slightly. Rub palms together till warm and lightly place centre of the palms over the eyeballs. Focus the mind on the palms. Breathe naturally for two minutes (a count of about one hundred).

Therapeutic Functions:

- Activates the flow of energy qi and blood to the eyes.
- Relieves eye fatigue and heaviness in the head.
- Improves eyesight.
- Prevents/treats eye ailments.

Ear Exercise (耳功)

Application Figure 7

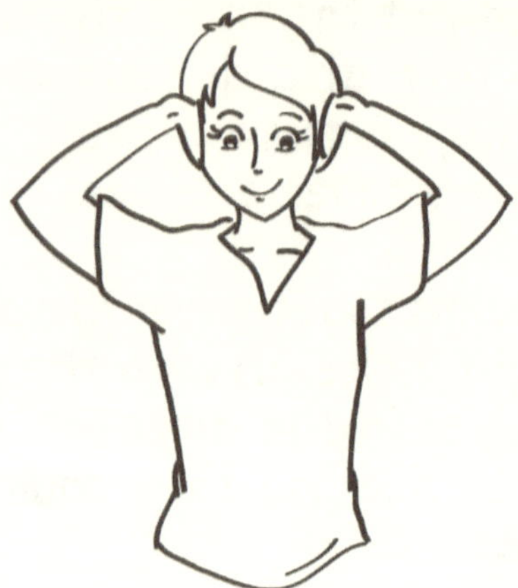

Press palms against the ears with fingers at the back of the head.

Massage and Acupressure Procedures:

1. Press the palms against the ears with the fingers at the back of the head. Place the index fingers onto the middle fingers. Flick the index fingers downward 18 times. (The sound of drum-beating can be heard.)

2. Place the palms against the ears. Press tightly and release quickly. Upon releasing, say aloud the word *hei* 9-18 times.

3. Place the bottom of the palms on top of the ears. Push the palms 9-18 times all the way down the auricles.

4. Rub the sides of the ears with the index and middle fingers 9-18 times.

5. Use the thumb and index finger to press on the ear lobes. Count 9-18 times.

Therapeutic Functions:

- Activates the flow of energy *qi* and blood to the external and internal ear.
- Calms the nerves.
- Improves hearing.
- Prevents/treats tinnitus (ringing in the ears) and deafness.

Chest Exercise (胸功)

Application Figure 8

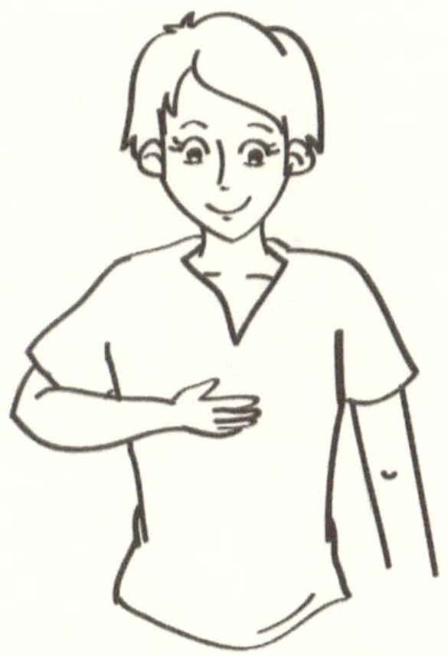

Push palm across the median line of the chest left to right, then from right to left

Massage and Acupressure Procedures:

1. Place the palm on the chest and rub in a circular motion 9-18 times.

2. Push the right and left palm alternately across the median line of the chest 9-18 times. Move the right palm from left to right. Then use the left palm to push from right to left.

Therapeutic Functions:

- Regulates the flow of *qi* energy.
- Relieves tightness of the chest.
- Relieves frequent yawning.
- Prevents/treats coughing.

Abdomen Exercise (腹功)

Application Figure 9

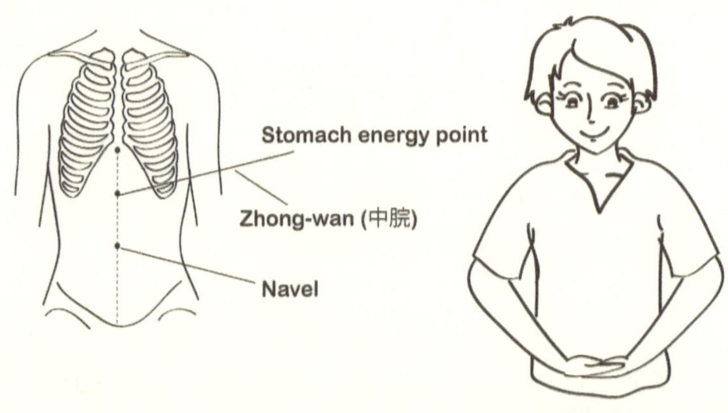

Massage and Acupressure Procedures:

1. Place the centre of the palms, one on top the other, on the navel. Press and knead in a clockwise motion to a count of nine from the navel up to the stomach, then in a counter-clockwise motion back to the navel to another count of nine.

2. Place the palms (facing upwards,) one on top the other, below the lower abdomen. Jerk the lower abdomen upwards 9-18 times.

3. Place the palms, one on top the other, on the navel and breathe calmly to nurture the dantian elixir field for two minutes (a count of about one hundred).

Therapeutic Functions:

- Replenishes the loss of *qi* in the dantian elixir field.
- Regulates the flow of *qi* and blood to the digestive system.
- Strengthens the functions of the spleen and stomach.
- Prevents/treats gastric pain, ulcers, yawning, and belching

Kidney Exercise (肾功)

Application Figure 10

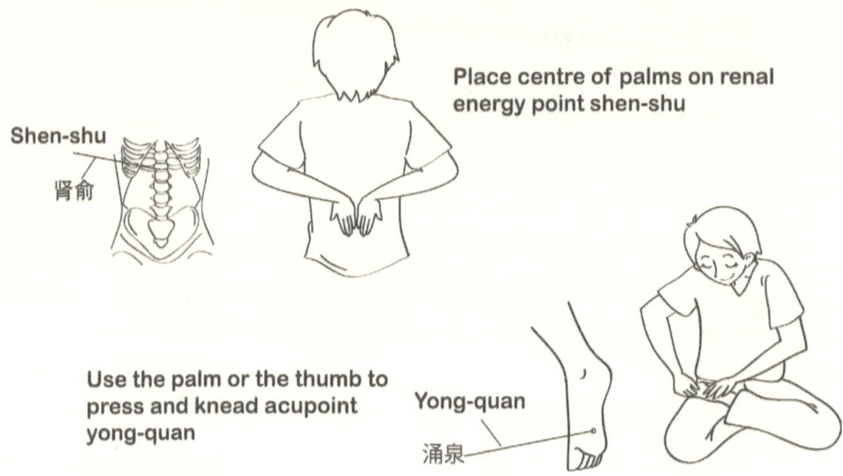

Massage and Acupressure Procedures:

1. Use the left and right palms to slap alternately 9-18 times on the navel and *ming-men* (命门) acupoints.

2. Warm the palms. Place the centre of palms on the renal acupoint *shen-shu* (肾俞) (around lumbar 4-5) for a while. Take a deep breath, then push the palms up and down, from the renal point to the sacrum with normal breathing. Push 9-18 times or more.

3. With arms akimbo and using the waist as the pivot, turn in circles from left to right 9-18 times, then from right to left 9-18 times.

4. Stand or sit from thirty seconds to two minutes with hands cupped over the navel.

5. Place the centre of the palm on the arch of the left foot over acupoint *yong-quan* (涌泉). Press and knead on it 9-18 times. Repeat the same on the right foot.

Therapeutic Functions:

- Activate flow of qi and blood into the kidneys.
- Tone muscles of the waist.
- Prevent/treat lumbago, weak knee and frequent urination.
- Relieve insomnia

Points to Remember

- Stand or sit as desired.
- Do not massage after a heavy meal. Neither do we massage when feeling hungry.
- Do not massage when under medical treatment.
- Use the palms of hands, the knuckles, and the fleshy part of the thumbs and fingers as your tools. Avoid using finger nails or other hard objects.
- All acupoints are painful when pressure is applied on them. If there is no pain from where the finger is resting, move a little to the left or right, top or bottom until pain is felt.

Before You Begin:

- Lower your eyelids.
- Relax by breathing naturally and gently with hands cupped over the navel.

During the Massage:

- Get rid of stray thoughts by directing '*mind-will (意念*') to the spot being massaged.
- To knead (rub) in a circular motion means doing one round of massage clockwise and then another round in counter-clockwise direction.
- Apply light, steady pressure when pressing, kneading, or pushing the acupoints.
- During acupressure, inhale at the acupoint. Exhale when applying the pressure. Always breathe gently.
- Do not rush through the exercise. Being slow and steady gains better results.

At the End of the Massage:

- Relax by sitting or standing calmly with hands cupped over the navel.

SELF-AID AT A GLANCE

Ailments	Affected *Qi* Channels	Self-Aid Tools	
		The Exercise Regimens in Mobile Qigong	**Massage with Acupressure**
Abdomen (lower) tense and cold	Heart, small intestine pericardium	Harmonise yin-yang *qi*, heart, triple heater	Abdomen
Allergy	Triple heater	Harmonise yin-yang *qi*, triple heater	Chest, abdomen
Anaemic	Gall bladder, stomach	Harmonise yin-yang *qi*, liver, spleen	Abdomen
Appetite (no craving for food)	Liver, spleen, Stomach	Harmonise yin-yang *qi*, liver, spleen	Abdomen
Asthma	Lungs	Harmonise yin-yang *qi*, lung, triple heater	Nose
Blood pressure (abnormal)	Pericardium, triple heater	Harmonise yin-yang *qi*, heart, triple heater	Head, chest
Blood circulation (poor)	Small intestine, spleen, stomach	Harmonise yin-yang *qi*, heart, spleen, triple heater	Chest, abdomen

Body system (easily poisoned)	Liver	Harmonise yin-yang *qi*, liver, triple heater	Abdomen
Chest, arms, and upper abdomen (tight)	Lungs, large intestine, triple heater	Harmonise yin-yang *qi*, lungs, triple heater	Chest, abdomen
Constipation	Gall bladder, small intestine, large intestine, kidneys	Harmonise yin-yang *qi*, liver, heart, lungs, kidneys	Teeth, chest, abdomen, kidney. **Diet:** Psyllium husks; fibre fruits like apples, pears, bananas; vegetables like Chinese spinach, broccoli, cabbage. Drink lots of water
Common cold or influenza (prone to)	Stomach, lungs, triple heater	Harmonise yin-yang *qi*, spleen, lungs, triple heater	Nape of neck, nose, chest, abdomen
Coughing (with or without phlegm)	Liver, gall bladder, lungs	Harmonise yin-yang *qi*, liver, lungs	Nose, chest
Digestion (poor)	Spleen, small intestine	Harmonise yin-yang *qi*, heart, spleen	Tongue, abdomen
Dizziness	Triple heater	Harmonise yin-yang *qi*, triple heater	Head, neck, face

Ears (deafness, tinnitus, pain)	Small intestine, kidneys, liver, spleen	Harmonise yin-yang *qi*, heart, kidneys	Ears, chest, kidney
Eyes (heavy, tired, pain)	Gall bladder, small intestine, urinary bladder	Harmonise yin-yang *qi*, liver, heart, kidneys	Eye, chest, kidney
Face (lacklustre)	Spleen, kidneys, liver	Harmonise yin-yang *qi*, spleen, kidneys, liver	Face, abdomen, kidneys
Fatigue	Liver, stomach, heart, kidneys	Harmonise yin-yang *qi*, liver, spleen, heart, kidneys	Chest, abdomen, kidneys
Fever (without cause)	Liver	Harmonise yin-yang *qi*, liver	Abdomen
Gastric (chronic pain)	Gall bladder, stomach,	Harmonise yin-yang *qi*, liver, spleen	Abdomen
Headache	Gall bladder, small intestine, large intestine, urinary bladder, pericardium	Harmonise yin-yang *qi*, liver, heart, lung, kidneys triple heater	Head, nape of neck, face, kidneys
Hip (fatigue)	Small intestine	Harmonise yin-yang *qi*, heart	chest
Insomnia (not enough sleep)	Kidneys	Harmonise yin-yang *qi*, kidney	Nose, kidney

Itchy skin	Large intestine, triple heater	Harmonise yin-yang *qi*, lungs, triple heater	Chest, abdomen, kidney
Legs (heavy, tired)	Gall bladder, small intestine, urinary bladder,	Harmonise yin-yang *qi*, liver, heart, kidney	Chest, kidney
Menstrual cycle (abnormal)	Small intestine Kidneys	Harmonise yin-yang *qi*, heart, kidney	Kidney, chest
Mouth (bitter taste)	Gall bladder	Harmonise yin-yang *qi*, liver	Teeth and tongue
Mouth (sticky and dry)	Spleen	Harmonise yin-yang *qi*, spleen	Teeth and tongue
Nails (cracked)	Kidney	Harmonise yin-yang *qi*, kidneys	Kidney
Neck, shoulders and arms (pain)	Triple heater, lungs	Harmonise yin-yang *qi*, lung, triple heater	Nape of neck Chest, kidney
Nose (running) (congestion)	Large intestine, triple heater	Harmonise yin-yang *qi*, lungs, triple heater	Nose
Palpitations	Heart, pericardium	Harmonise yin-yang *qi*, heart, triple heater	Chest
Rash	Triple heater	Harmonise yin-yang *qi*, triple heater	Abdomen, kidney

Rib cage (pain)	Gall bladder, triple heater	Harmonise yin-yang *qi*, liver, triple heater	Abdomen, kidney
Saliva (lack of secretion)	Small intestine, spleen	Harmonise yin-yang *qi*, heart, spleen	Tongue
Shortness of breath	Lungs	Harmonise yin-yang *qi*, lungs. (Use *hu* (呼) to blow out the air, not the character formula *si* (四.)	**Remedy:** Inhale through the nose, exhale through the mouth, saying the word ***soong*** (松) and sinking it down to the navel. (Do six times.)
Shoulders (tense, stiff, pain)	Liver, gall bladder, heart, lungs, urinary bladder, spleen, and stomach	Harmonise yin-yang *qi*, liver, heart, lungs, spleen, kidneys	Chest, abdomen, kidney
Sinus (cold in the head)	Gall bladder, large intestine, urinary bladder	Harmonise yin-yang *qi*, liver, lungs, kidneys	Nape of neck, nose, kidneys
Spine (pain)	Spleen	Harmonise yin-yang *qi*, spleen, triple heater	Abdomen, kidney (do only procedures 1 & 2)

Note:

To begin, always stand or sit for two minutes, breathing gently to calm the mind and emotions.

During treatment, we must not take the wrong food. For example, if we are suffering from stomach ulcer, we should avoid taking raw, cold, and pungent food that could irritate the stomach. If we have hypertension, we should maintain a healthy mood and avoid being overly excited. Only by such means can self-aid be effective. Always remember to consult the doctor first and then take the medicine prescribed. When you have recovered, make use of self-aid to keep fit.

Epilogue

I have put twenty-six years of practice into Tranquil Qigong (Meditation), Mobile Qigong, and ten years into Massage with Acupressure. These three forms, introduced in the book, can safely be catalogued as the source of my health. As readers will have noticed, I only make claims to the therapeutic effects as felt by my body without giving any rational explanation in a scientific way for any of the claims. Those who have gone through many years of Qigong practice will understand that feelings and experiences like those of general ease, calm, restfulness, quiescence, tranquillity, and the tingling sensation in the skin are just too difficult for anyone to grasp or comprehend by explanation. This is much so when the degree of beneficial effects varies from individual to individual because of different physical conditions and different practicing techniques. Two testimonies written by my students are printed for readers to understand individual differences in experience with Qigong practice. The testimonies also reveal my students' absolute confidence, trust, and belief in the positive effects of Qigong practice on their ailments and improvement to their health. This is clearly "love through knowing and understanding."

Over the years, much has been said by people from different walks of life about the effectiveness of Qigong as a healthcare therapy. In order that the basic quality of Qigong practice is not misinterpreted, the following paragraphs hope to provide an understanding to the true nature of Qigong.

1. Every one of us is an individual. Eventual results from our practices depend on our own physical, emotional, and mental conditions. Each of us has different inherent make-up and lifestyle—our diet, our habits, our living and work environment, and the stress and tension that may be causing us mental exhaustion. Under such variable conditions, each one of us will experience differently the energy *qi* flow and circulation. Some may feel the flow and circulation of *qi* sooner (in a few weeks), while others may feel it later (in a few months). Some may feel warm, while others may feel cool. Some have pain sensations, while others feel pins and needles. I sometimes sensed prickly pain during practice. My master used to say it was a message the body sent to the mind. It could either be that healing was taking place or that an ailment had surfaced.

2. When illness befalls us, Qigong practice does not stand alone. It complements medical recommendations given by doctors. All the exercises given in this book are not to be

taken as substitutes for medical advice. We must always consult the doctor whenever problems or ailments persist for more than three days.

On one occasion, pain around my lower abdomen was quite severe and was accompanied by a heavy head and tired eyes. I consulted the doctor and found I had stones in the gall bladder.

3. Qigong takes time, and you must take pains to develop it into an effective therapy. Not everyone experiences the same therapeutic effects. Much depends on how much time and effort is being put into its practice. We must not chase results but let things take their natural course.

4. Qigong is like cooking a meal. The cook can have all the right ingredients, but if they are not used proportionately or cooked with the correct timing and temperature, the flavour will be lost. Qigong may have all the techniques, but if they are not applied appropriately to individual needs or practiced accurately in accordance to the nature of its form, the therapeutic effect will go astray.

5. Given that wrong diet, overeating, physical, mental, and emotional stress, or environmental conditions could upset our healthiness, to experience good therapeutic results we must

develop a routine. Practise regularly every day, if unable, three or four times a week. Be constant with the same style of Qigong rather than switching styles from one school to another.

6. Be careful not to be overstrained from doing too many different styles of the Qigong exercises that are available in the market. Obvious warning signs that you are overdoing it are headache, excessive fatigue after exercising, tired eyes, tightness in the chest, or depression.

In conclusion, Qigong practice is disciplining the mind to wipe out vexing passions and worrying thoughts. Only then can we help ourselves to treat chronic health problems when they arise or prevent them from getting worse. Even when we have no ailments, Qigong practice maintains our health to avoid having diseases in the future.

Every one of us can form our own opinion as to how we wish to practise the art. However, there has to be a time when we must be prepared to accept a guided, disciplined system—a system that may require us to change our lifestyle.

Testimony

A Testimony by Claudia Heck

How Qigong Helped My Recovery and Health

I was first introduced to Traditional Chinese Qigong in 2005 by my friend Madam Chan Siok Fong, who subsequently became my master.

I had just been discharged from hospital after liver surgery to remove a liver abscess caused by a bacteria called kelbsiella.

Suffice to say that I was weak, void of energy and stamina.

Madam Chan patiently and systematically taught me the necessary Qigong movements as follows:

- She first taught me the harmonizing and lung movements to clear the water that was still in my lungs at the point of discharge from the hospital

- This was followed by the liver movement to strengthen my liver and help in its recovery.

- When she felt that I was ready, she taught me the rest of the movements to complete the set for holistic health.

During a routine check-up at the hospital at the end of the first month after my discharge, the doctor was surprised that the water in my lungs had "evaporated" and I did not require a procedure to draw the water from my lungs.

By the tenth month, the surgeon again expressed interest at how my liver was "biologically full" again. Of course, it was smaller in size than the original, but it was 100% "regrown" in medical terms. The surgeon asked me what I was doing besides taking medication.

I told him that I was practising Traditional Chinese Qigong.

He said he didn't know or understand Qigong but that it appeared to have helped me tremendously. Patients who had some fifteen per cent of their liver cut away would normally regrow it to "full" size within 12-18 months, but mine was "full" by the tenth month. He even joked that I should perhaps get my Qigong master to teach his other liver patients.

One can understand from this why I loudly proclaim the benefits of Traditional Chinese Qigong and practise it faithfully.

Last but not least, I thank Madam Chan for her patience and unfailing guidance in helping me regain my health and energy.

Claudia Heck

A Testimony by Chan Jing Oi

How Qigong Helped in My Recovery

In the past I never paid much attention to exercise. Then in 1997 I fell sick after two successive bouts of cold. I felt very weak. I had difficulty climbing the stairs and was having cold sweats and cold hands. At that time, I was unable to take any MSG, so I could never eat out. My hands would swell even after eating a piece of *char siew pau* (dumpling)

At that time, I met my niece Chan Siok Fong for the first time. We had never met before because we used to live in different parts of Malaysia, and I had never known previously that she had moved to Singapore.

After our meeting, I became more health-conscious. Siok Fong then taught me the full set of Traditional Chinese Qigong, consisting of meditation (tranquil Qigong) and *da yan liu zi gong* (mobile Qigong). She gave me lessons twice a week until I could practise each exercise regimen systematically on my own. I painstakingly disciplined myself to practise every day. After a few months of regular and constant practice, amazingly I was gradually able to eat restaurant-cooked and hawker-cooked food. My hands no longer swelled. My appetite improved, and I began to feel stronger. Moreover, I now seldom catch cold.

Years later, even after having been on dialysis treatment for eight years, and despite my age of eighty-three, I am still the healthiest patient at the dialysis centre among those between sixty and eighty-five years of age.

I am always grateful to Siok Fong for giving me this new lease of life. This is my advice to all my dear friends: "Practice Traditional Chinese Qigong whenever you have the chance. Do not wait until you are too old."

Chan Jing Oi

www.ingramcontent.com/pod-product-compliance
Lightning Source LLC
Chambersburg PA
CBHW020517290526
45786CB00002B/640

* 9 7 8 1 4 8 1 7 8 7 5 8 1 *